DAY 6: BEYOND 1

Refreshed & Revised for Toda
(Second Edition 2020)

KAYE BAILEY

.

Day 6: Beyond the 5 Day Pouch Test

Refreshed & Revised for Today's Discerning WLS Community (Second Edition 2020)

The health content in Day 6: Beyond the 5 Day Pouch Test is intended to inform, not prescribe, and is not meant to be a substitute for the advice and care of a qualified health-care professional. The author and publisher disclaim any liability arising directly or indirectly from the use of this book.

A LIVINGAFTERWLS PUBLICATION
Proudly serving the healthy weight management and
weight loss surgery community since 2005.

TABLE OF CONTENTS

Nutritional Analysis: Every effort has been made to check the accuracy of the nutritional information that appears with each recipe. However, because numerous variables account for a wide range of values for certain foods, nutritive analyses in this book should be considered approximate. Different results may be obtained by using different nutrient databases and different brand-name products.

Serving Size: For purposes of continuity recipe serving size and nutrient values are calculated and measured on the Daily Values standard for a 2,000 calorie/day diet for adults, developed by the Food and Drug Administration (FDA). It is understood that people who have undergone a restrictive bariatric surgical procedure will eat less than the standard serving size, and that people with different bariatric procedures will eat different volumes of food per serving. Please use the serving size and nutrient values provided as the baseline factor from which to calculate and adjust your specific and unique dietary intake.

INTRODUCTION:

Twenty years ago I "Arrived" on September 13, 1999 in San Diego California exactly one month to the day after Carnie Wilson put weight loss surgery (WLS) on the map. It was at once one of the most exciting and frightening things I have ever done. Back in the day the Internet was just taking hold and my research was sketchy at best. I knew I wanted WLS because I grew up in a culture of obesity and felt it was my only solution. As I learned about surgery there was a procedure called laparoscopic gastric bypass that was being done by few surgeons, but with great success. The surgeon nearest me was 1,500 miles away in San Diego.

My pre-op consultation was done by telephone, and would you believe, snail mail? Even the pre-op psychiatric examine was pre-historic. I sat with a counselor at a local do-it-yourself "mental health" office and he knew nothing about weight management or bariatric counseling. However, he did confirm that I did not have the tendency to maim small children and it was unlikely I would become an ax murderer. What a relief to learn that. I was approved for surgery.

We went to San Diego and met the surgeon and staff on Friday, and I had surgery on Monday. I don't recall much about that day. I remember feeling embarrassed lying on the preparation table, my enormous belly exposed for cleansing by a stranger. I remember feeling frightened, but calm with a total acceptance that gastric bypass surgery was the best decision for me. I remember the anesthesiologist, a young beautiful petite woman. Then I went to sleep.

I woke up nauseated, an unpleasant reaction to anesthesia. I didn't have my glasses, so things were blurry, particularly the flowers from my husband. And I can remember a push-button device that helped me sleep. Later that night I realized I was not yet smaller. In fact, my stomach was bloated and sore. In my drug induced confusion, I was convinced the surgeon had mistakenly done the wrong operation because I was getting bigger, not smaller.

The day after surgery my surgeon visited me, taught me to drink tiny sips of water from a paper cup much like a sacrament cup. He patted my hand and told me I was going to do just fine. I remember walking around the hospital hallway. I remember a female nurse bathing me. I remember a good-looking male nurse: he didn't bathe me. I remember drinking some nasty liquid chalk and getting an X-ray to confirm my stomach had been whacked, stapled and bypassed. I remember the super-sized wheelchair and being embarrassed that I fit in it snugly.

I remember being discharged from the hospital to spend the next several days in a motel room because we had traveled a great distance for my "last resort" surgery. I was neither ill nor well. Those recovery days held me captive: An indeterminate limbo. I watched reruns, mostly old westerns, on a fuzzy-picture television. The sofa at the motor lodge was scratchy. My husband and I went on outings each day, little drives around a strange town. He emptied my surgical drain for me. I thought it was disgusting.

On Thursday of the second week Leslie, the darling nurse and counselor, herself a WLS patient, removed my drain. Finally, we could go home. She asked me the Four Rules and I repeated them to her. She told me, "Take advantage of this window of opportunity. Learn everything you can. If you don't learn early to follow the rules and take care of yourself, you can regain this weight."

Starry eyed and hopeful we packed ourselves in the car and headed for home. Almost 1,500 miles later we pulled into the driveway of home sweet home. My fabulous husband said to me, "Welcome to your new life – You Have Arrived."

And I was all alone, 1,500 miles from help. All my consults were done by telephone, so I had to find my own way. My information binder was a constant companion and I followed the Four Rules without waver. By late 2000 I was at my low weight and thrilled. I was also exhausted and slept nearly that whole summer. The trauma of surgery and massive weight loss had exhausted my system. My emotions were out of control too. I've since learned that because estrogen is stored in fat cells that when fat is lost quickly estrogen levels become imbalanced. On my one-year "*Arrivalversary*" we returned to San Diego where my center proclaimed me a success.

Year two was a whirl for me. No longer able to binge on food I binged on clothes. Never having shopped at the "little people" stores I was drunk over shoes and skirts and slacks and handbags. I can recall crying: crying like a baby, when I could try things on, and they fit and I looked good. I also remember seeing my reflection and wondering, "Who is that?" It was also in the second year that my husband took hundreds of pictures of me. I wasn't afraid of the camera any longer.

With my confidence in place year three brought a testing of the rules and I made love to my first slider food: graham crackers and coffee after work. Lots of graham crackers and coffee. As you can guess I gained some weight back, a couple of pounds at first. It was easy to ignore because this was my strongest year of physical fitness; I the gain to an increase in muscle weight.

By year four I was sick of being all about weight loss surgery and just wanted to be normal again without worrying about every bite, every calorie and every protein gram. I stopped talking about weight loss surgery and left my online groups so I could be normal. At year five post-surgery I was a "normal" 20 pounds overweight I despaired. Why did I go through weight loss surgery and cosmetic reconstruction just to gain weight? It was also during this time LivingAfterWLS was evolving first with a blog followed by a website and eventually LivingAfterWLS online community, "The Neighborhood" which is now shuttered. My first book of weight loss surgery self-help "The 5 Day Pouch Test Owner's Manual" was published in 2007 with followed by several titles for the weight loss surgery lifestyle.

I came to a calm realization in year six that I will always have the disease of morbid obesity and it is my responsibility to keep it in remission with diet, exercise and self-nurturing. I also learned that a back-to-basics approach was needed and began experimenting with what became the 5 Day Pouch Test.

The first edition of Day 6 marked my 10-year *"Arrivalversary"*. I was fighting that wicked back-n-forth 20 pounds again but vowed that no matter what the scale said, no matter what the size of my jeans I would daily, "Stop for a moment and look where I am: I Have Arrived."

That edition contained a collection of information gathered in the first ten years post-gastric bypass. Remarkably, much of that information holds true a decade later as I mark twenty years. As I begin my third decade of "LivingAfterWLS" I offer this updated Second Edition that includes the best of the first edition with several new features relevant in today's world of LivingAfterWLS.

New and Noteworthy in 2020:

Obesity Medicine: In 2013 The American Medical Association (AMA) made headlines when its governing body adopted a policy that recognized obesity as a disease requiring a range of medical interventions to advance obesity treatment and prevention. Slowly, but steadily, a paradigm shift is taking place making it possible for increased obesity research and funding, improved obesity counseling and education, the FDA approval of pharmaceutical treatments, coverage for obesity-related service by Medicaid, Medicare, Affordable Care Act, and many private health insurance plans. This designation, though not without controversy, makes it possible for those suffering from the disease obesity to work with the medical community in the treatment and management of a dire health condition that prematurely ends 300,000 lives each year in the United States.

Typically, obese patients avoid discussing obesity, diet, and lifestyle factors with our general care doctors because it is uncomfortable. Too often, we are made to feel inadequate, foolish, or perhaps ashamed. It is much more comfortable to seek weight loss solutions from consumer sources rather than our healthcare providers. Historically the insurance industry has enabled this discomfort by failing to provide coverage for obesity thus making clear the problem is the fault of the patient without considering the medical diagnosis. I know I believed that because my health insurance denied all obesity claims then the obesity must be my fault, a personal moral flaw, not a health problem.

The tide has turned in the last five years and providing valid care and specialized treatment is the new standard for many health care providers and their affiliates. The current fact-based data supports the necessity of patient and doctor responsibility in managing this disease and medical professionals are listening. This designation empowered the American

Board of Obesity Medicine (ABOM), chartered in 2011, to advance the field of specialized obesity medicine, subsequently leading to a corps of certified Obesity Medicine Physician.

Obesity medicine is now established as the one of the fastest growing fields in medicine. The ABOM reported the number of board-certified obesity physicians exceeds 2,650 in the U.S. and Canada (March 2018). "The rapid growth of obesity medicine certification highlights the fact that physicians now recognize they need tools to help treat the many patients they see with obesity," said ABOM Executive Director Dana Brittan. "The certification process helps provide those tools, and the certification itself sends a signal to other physicians and the public that there are doctors ready, willing and able to support patients with obesity."

This ABOM certification identifies a "physician with expertise in the sub-specialty of obesity medicine. This sub-specialty requires competency in and a thorough understanding of the treatment of obesity and the genetic, biologic, environmental, social, and behavioral factors that contribute to obesity." ABOM designates board certified physicians as "Diplomats" and their growing corps includes internists, family physicians, pediatricians), endocrinologists, obstetricians, gynecologists, gastroenterologists and surgeons, along with numerous other specialists. Visit the American Board of Obesity Medicine website to find a physician in your area certified in obesity medicine: https://www.abom.org/

The Weight Loss Consumer: As early as the 1950's Americans have sought weight loss solutions in the commercial market abundant with programs, pills, meals and deals guaranteed to promote fast dramatic weight loss. In fact, the U.S. weight loss market is worth a record $66 billion at the end of 2017. Trends indicate more of our dieting dollars will be spent for medical solutions rather than retail solutions. We can credit the obesity as a disease designation for this consumer shift. Not to be left behind, the weight loss retail market is changing favorably to bring us improved products known as clean meals or clean meal replacements. More health and weight loss products are available from traditional food producers thus lowering the cost and increasing the variety of options available at neighborhood supermarkets. For example, I am thrilled to find a protein-fortified oatmeal by Quaker at my local market. The Quaker oatmeal, nutritionally compatible with weight loss specialty products is about .60 cents a serving. The specialized bariatric high protein oatmeal averages $2 per serving. We can be encouraged knowing this trend will continue and we will be able to enjoy food that supports our bariatric lifestyle and goals without breaking the bank.

Not Your Grandma's Diet Pills: The diet pill industry has benefitted from the 2013 designation of obesity as a disease. Increased research funding in pharmacology has facilitated a new emphasis promoting the inclusion of anti-obesity medications (AOMs) in the overall treatment of obesity. Increasingly pharmaceuticals are prescribed to work in tandem with bariatric surgical procedures. Speaking before the Government Accountability Office in July 2018 Wendy Scinta, president of the Obesity Medicine Association, presented compelling data supporting medical weight loss. She noted recent research on metabolic adaptation supports the medication and medical management of obesity. In fact, there are presently 128 obesity drugs in active development signaling that pharmacotherapy will play a role in the future of obesity treatment. In the future AOMs are likely to be included in the post-surgical protocol for many patients with the expectation of improved weight loss results.

You will find a 2018 scholarly review of weight loss medications in the Appendix. Having fact-based understanding of these medications is essential when working with our health care providers in the ongoing management of obesity.

Additionally, throughout the text of Day 6 you will find information to serve you well in the weight loss surgery odyssey well into the next decade.

Thanks for joining me here in Day 6: Beyond the 5 Day Pouch Test. This book is divided in three parts: Part I: DAY 6 DIET; Part II: Day 6 Fundamentals and Part III: Cooking with Kaye. Please pay careful attention to Chapter 1 of DAY 6 DIET: it is the most important chapter you will read in this book and I guarantee it will change the way you feel about the word DIET forever. In Chapters 2 and 3 of Part I we review the Four Rules and the 5 Day Pouch Test: both key lessons in our long-term weight loss surgery lifestyle. Part II covers the fundamentals of Day 6 including the DAY 6 DIET Basics and DAY 6 DIET Intelligence. Finally, we complete the picture with a workable embraceable Day 6 plan: Putting it All Together. In Part III you are invited to join me in my kitchen as we prepare some of my favorite recipes and I explain why they work well for my family and me in this LivingAfterWLS lifestyle.

Other Updates. In addition to the big topic updates to this Second Edition you will notice more subtle changes as recipes were updated for 2020 and citable information was updated with the latest findings. It was an enlightening experience for me realize how much has changed since the First Edition in 2009. I think the future is bright for the WLS population. Awareness about the true nature of obesity is growing. The more we treat this as a medical issue that must be managed medically the more progress we will enjoy. I'm certain the one thing that will not change is the attention and effort maintaining a healthy weight requires. We signed up for life and now, marking 20 years, I'm starting to understand what that truly means. Enjoy these updates and settle back for the life-long journey we are taking together.

PART I: DAY 6 DIET

"Don't forget that being thin is a life management skill. It is normal to experience setbacks and periods of feeling defeated. But in the future when you turn 40 or 50 or 60 at a healthy weight it won't be by accident, because aging well is not an accident. It's the gift that those who care deeply give to themselves. It will be because you planned and honed your skills at weight management." --Dr. Stephen P. Gullo

CHAPTER 1: LET'S HAVE TEA

This is the most important chapter you will read in this book. So please, set aside some time, find a quiet place. Make yourself comfortable and join me in an important conversation. Because the thoughts I share here will make a difference in how you manage your fork, your thoughts, and your weight loss surgery for the rest of your life. If you were to sit on my sofa and ask, "Kaye, tell me your secrets after ten years," this is what I would tell you, over a cup of warm ginger lemon tea, of course.

Let's begin with a confession: I love the word diet.

For decades society has whored the word diet until it has become an ugly stepsister loathed by fat and thin alike. In fact, many of us became obese by following the latest "fad diet". You know them all. But did you know that the word diet, a noun, is simply defined as the foods and beverages a person eats and drinks? More historically, diet is a Greek word that means "mode of life," especially one prescribed by a physician that includes the regulation of eating habits. The earliest recorded English definition of diet is "food, daily provisions," and that is the current correct usage.

Yet in our modern civilization we have adulterated the word to mean extreme dietary restriction, odd food combining, punishment, false promises, and fleeting hope. By the time we pursue and undergo weight loss surgery we often declare our emancipation from dieting forever. I know I did. Diets had failed and I would no longer be in the servitude of the diet industry.

Nearly 20 years after weight loss surgery I am not on a diet and I have not returned to dieting servitude. But food, my daily provisions, are my diet and to them I am true.

Let me explain. In my obese life I was either dieting or I was not dieting. The dieting meant I was following a plan, and several times I enjoyed the euphoria of weight loss that others noticed and complimented. But the diets were so oddly structured, as quick-fix diets usually are, that as soon as I stopped following them, and went back to normal, the inescapable weight gain occurred. It was only a few short pounds from euphoria to anguish. This pattern repeated countless times and I learned that dieting does cause weight loss. Not dieting, or going back to normal, causes weight gain.

When I was preparing for weight loss surgery, I learned about the Four Rules and, still suffering chronic dieting mentality, believed that I would only need to follow the Four Rules until I achieved goal weight. Then I could get back to normal. At a support group session before having surgery I heard a gastric bypass patient say, "I can eat anything I want, just less of it," with a big hearty belly laugh. Naturally, I assumed this was true, that I would be able to eat anything I wished, and the tool would do the work. I would never ever have to follow a diet again. What a relief.

For a long time, I thought I was the only one foolish enough to think I would never have to diet again after surgery. But now I know that most of us think we will never have to follow a diet again; surgery will cure us of that.

The truth is, in order to make our tool work we must mindfully follow a diet. Not just during weight loss, but for the rest of our lives.

Please, have a sip of your tea, and let's continue our conversation. I have a request.

I ask you to consider your relationship with the word diet. It is a perfectly good word that quickly communicates a message. Simple words function well as I realized when looking at a road map. The title of the road map was

"Geographical Rendering of Highways with Topographical & Historical Features." The word "map" did not appear anywhere on the document. Yet when Jim asked me, "May I see the map?" I knew exactly what he was asking for. Map was the best word to describe the tool he wanted to use to plan a route from one destination to the next. Sometimes the lowliest word is best.

So it goes with the word diet. I have been writing about weight loss surgery and dieting for years. Over that time I have tried to use trendy expressions in lieu of the dreaded "D-Word" such as way-of-eating, healthy eating, high-protein consumption, WLS-way-of-eating and a few others that are just plain silly. Consequently, in working on this Day 6 book I was compelled to ditch the cutesy synonyms and make amends with our ugly stepsister "diet" and let her know that we love her for the simple natural beauty she is. We do not despise the ugly whore our society has made her to be.

I offer this, Day 6 DIET Creed, so we may build a better relationship with food, our daily provisions, and our mode of life:

DAY 6 DIET

DAILY *adjective*: for each day

INTELLIGENT *adjective*: consistent with reason and intellect: consequent, logical, rational, reasonable

EATING *verb*: to consume food: to take or have a meal

TRIUMPHS *verb*: to feel and express uplifting joy over success and victory

DAILY INTELLIGENT EATING TRIUMPHS

It turns out our ugly stepsister is a natural beauty of extraordinary simplicity. When you read it like that you just want to make DIET part of your day. It is not the same dirty word nagging easy rapid weight loss from the supermarket tabloids.

Let's discuss each word in our acronym DIET, beyond the definition. First, may I pour you another cup of tea?

Daily. Perhaps the best-known reminder that we must partake food daily is from the Holy Bible, *"Give us this day our daily bread."* (Matthew 6:11) While that is a prayer of thanks it is also a reminder that to nurture our bodies, we must provide food. That means every new day we have an opportunity to make right our nutritional wellness. We have at least three chances daily to feed our body the things it needs so it can give back to us sturdy bones and strong muscles, healthy lungs, clear eyes, and a sharp mind. How exciting that every single day of our life we have the opportunity enrich our life and health with nutritional generosity. I get goose bumps just thinking about my next opportunity to build healthier me.

Intelligent. I love this part of DIET because the weight loss surgery community is notoriously gluttonous for intelligence. Before surgery we are near-hysterical researchers. After surgery we are constant knowledge seekers and question askers. Why, here you are with this book in hand, seeking intelligence. So naturally it stands to reason that when it comes to our DIET we will act with reason and intellect in a consequent, logical, rational, and reasonable manner. Good for you. Our inclination to pursue knowledge and learning is well served by this part of DIET.

We have only covered two of our four words and already you get to treat your body well and behave intelligently every day. I see you smiling. I thought you might grow fond of our new friend DIET.

Eating. Here is another favorite part of this acronym: Eating! Now that we are prepared to make intelligent dietary choices each day we get to the good part, eating. Based on your personal diet prescribed by your bariatric center you may eat three, four, or even five times a day. And since you made intelligent choices you will feel good physically and mentally. Making daily intelligent dietary choices gives us the freedom to enjoy eating without the mental anguish we all feel when we make poor unintelligent dietary choices.

Triumphs. Now for the celebration: You did it! As many times a day as you want you get to feel and express uplifting joy over success and victory! Now is the time to do the best happy dance ever. I'll join you. There is an abundance of joy in your heart: let it out! You have earned this triumph. You are a powerful intelligent individual and you have embraced DIET to make wise and careful choices to nurture health and contentment. The health and contentment you deserve to enjoy. Do the happy dance. Enjoy!

A little later in this book we will talk about the nitty- gritty of intelligent food choices, I have lots of ideas to share with you. But for now I hope you will stay with me and continue the conversation. There are some emotional issues we should discuss. And I am enjoying your company.

Let Freedom Ring. One of the most profound memories of my childhood is the Bicentennial pageant in 1976. I turned ten that year and I was the fattest child in my school class. But on a hot southern California July 4th this little fat girl carried a colonial flag in a patriotic pageant celebrating 200 years of national independence. It was the biggest thrill of my young life. I don't suppose I understood why tears fell from the faces of patriots who had just come home from across the sea fighting for a cause in which we did not believe. I don't suppose I understood the lump in my own throat when the marching band played the national anthem and I tried to sing along. I did know that I was an American, proud and lucky and strong. An American: Citizen of the most powerful nation in the world; resident in the land of the free and the home of the brave.

It was Independence Day.

Today I'm grown and have long since bid farewell to the Little Fat Girl. But come July 4th in a tiny Rocky Mountain town I'll stand on the sidewalk of Main Street, my hand over my heart, tears rolling down my cheeks unashamed when the old men from the American Legion carry our colors in the hometown parade. I'll cry for our country and for our servicemen and women. I'll swallow the lump in my throat and try to sing the words as the high school marching band plays the National Anthem and collectively, across this country, we salute our nation and celebrate our freedom.

And there is another Independence Day for which I am equally emotional: The Independence Day when surgical intervention released me from a lifetime of obesity. Because I know that without surgery I would have submitted to the disease that was slowly killing me pound by pound.

Even as my fidelity to country requires stewardship, so does my faithfulness to my health require stewardship. Patriotism cannot be benign or we lose the independence that engenders the patriotism in the first place. We cannot take our Independence lightly. Not national, not personal.

One thing that defines the LivingAfterWLS philosophy is the ownership and responsibility with which we manage our health. An often-quoted passage from the LivingAfterWLS Empowerment Philosophy reads: "LivingAfterWLS believes that success with weight loss surgery, and in life, can be found when we focus on inner strength rather than inner weakness. As recovering morbidly obese people we have often been made to feel weak for our illness. We are not weak. We have inner resources that make us beautiful unique beings with intelligence, talent, and love to share with the world." Harnessing this inner strength by way of personal responsibility is our stewardship. The reward for taking seriously our responsibility is improved health and wellness in the lifelong effort to manage the disease of obesity using our surgical weight loss tool.

The interesting thing about empowerment and independence is the more we take personal responsibility, the more we feel empowered and then we feel more independent. A feeling of independence, freedom of choice, gives us ownership in personal responsibility and accountability. It is a beautiful symbiotic circle of living.

Independence at the Price of Surrender. Over the years since surgery I have learned there is another independence that comes with surgery. Oddly enough, this independence comes at the price of surrender. We must surrender to the enemy, and guess what? The enemy is within. I have never met a post-WLS patient who at some point did not fight the rules and conditions that come with weight loss surgery, myself included. In fact, I made myself sick (vomiting or dumping) so many times in January 2002 that my calendar is covered in frowning faces. I did everything possible to prove that I controlled the surgery: the surgery did not control me. I was tired of following the rules, eating the same things, watching others eat things that I could or should not eat. And I was fighting a raging war against myself.

At the time I had a golden retriever named Louie who may have been conked on the head as a puppy: his dedication to fuzzy thinking was remarkable. He loved to play fetch. At playtime I tossed the tired old tennis ball with my best throw-like-a-girl pitch. Louie would dart after it and bring it back all wiggly and tail wagging. But he refused release the ball from his smiling slobbering mouth. I admonished, "Louie, I cannot throw a ball with a dog wrapped around it." And he would just keep wiggling and wagging, never releasing the ball. Game over.

It occurred to me that my little stomach pouch must have been saying the same thing to me: "I cannot keep you healthy with a rule-breaker wrapped around me." When I realized that the rules were there to protect me, to keep my tool and me healthy and in tiptop shape, I was able to surrender to them. I let go of the ball so the game could continue. See the metaphor here? Surrender is defined as the act of submitting or surrendering to the power of another: capitulation, submission. Usually surrender is a bad thing. But when we surrender to the terms and conditions, we agreed to by having weight loss surgery we make things a whole lot easier on ourselves. We find independence and freedom.

Never Forget! We agreed to the rules before surgery and we promised to follow them. We made this commitment willingly and wisely. The rules are our best protection against the behaviors that led us to morbid obesity and ultimately surgery. Why wouldn't we put our best effort forward to keep our word of honor in this battle for a better healthier life?

How are you feeling? Are you enjoying independence these days? Or are you fighting an inner battle? As hard I as try to keep the inner demons quiet, I occasionally get caught in a battle. It happens, please do not feel alone if you are struggling. Battles are won every day and you are a strong intelligent worthy person. And I am here with you.

Dropped Eggs Happen. As a lifelong person struggling with the disease of obesity the all-or-nothing mentality of falling off the wagon is something that continues to perplex me. Do you know what I'm talking about? I will have good intentions to have an omelet and tomato slices for breakfast but for some reason I chose instead to have a toasted bagel slathered with cream cheese. Naturally the high carbohydrate and high fat breakfast makes me feel sluggish and miserable, so I think, "To hell with it" and continue to make poor dietary choices the rest of the day. Now you know what I'm talking about, I see you nodding your head. (This still happens to me occasionally; I'll be honest with you.)

Years ago, in one of the many diet programs I was following, and I am not sure which it was, a counselor talked about dropped eggs as the theory applies to the scenario above. She asked if any of us, while in the kitchen baking, had accidentally dropped an egg on the floor. We all nodded yes. She then asked if we said, "To hell with it" and proceeded to drop the remaining eggs on the floor. We all nodded no, of course not! "Then why, when you drop the metaphorical diet egg do you say to hell with it and break the diet for the rest of the day?" This illustration is one I've never forgotten – I hope you find it useful as well.

Dropped eggs happen. We are human. We live in a difficult world. The next time you drop the proverbial diet egg visualize getting a paper towel, wiping up the spill and moving forward. Dropped eggs happen and a great deal of life and living is all about cleaning up messes.

Taking Care of Rocks. Each morning just before the sun illuminates the harsh Arizona desert an old man wearing beige dungarees and a cotton jacket rakes the rocks in his front yard. Many of the yards in Tucson are rocks: the harsh desert heat makes lush green lawns and shrubbery an environmental challenge at best. We passed the old man each morning on our walk and wondered why he was raking his rocks before dawn. He was methodical and intent. On the third morning my curiosity got the best of me. We stopped to speak to the old man of well-healed Japanese heritage.

After introductions I asked the old man, who was patting his brow with a handkerchief, "Why is it that you rake the rocks in your yard each morning?" Up close they looked like just rocks to me. He leaned on the handle of his rake silently looking at his rocks. At last he spoke, "Because, the garden is not finished."

Sensing the man was of few words and we were interrupting ritual we moved along on our morning walk. But I contemplated his words. The garden was not a living thing, how could it not be finished? Later I learned the Japanese rock garden (*Karensansui*) is a waterless garden made of gravel or sand that is raked, often into patterns that symbolize water, hills and mountains, and even plants. Zen certainly influenced the evolution of the Japanese rock garden. In fact, it is believed that early Zen priests practiced concentration and perfection while raking. Raking rocks is still a daily meditative ritual for many Japanese and practitioners of Zen. And so it was for the old man in the early Arizona dawn.

As I often do, I indulged my metaphorical fancies regarding gardening and our weight loss surgery journey. Like the old man we must rake our metaphorical weight loss surgery rocks each day because our body is not finished. And our body will not be finished until we stop breathing. Like the practice of Japanese rock gardening with rules and symbols, we in this weight loss surgery practice have rules to follow and symbols to respect. With careful daily attention our gardens, like the old man's, are a thing of beauty.

To my untrained eye the rock garden was just a yard of rocks. But to the thoughtful gardener it was a place of contemplation and meditation. It was a beautiful work in progress that would never be finished. And in this I learned that achieving perfection is not the goal, it is the quest for improvement and self-discovery, for the study, and learning that makes our gardens grow. As the garden is a work in progress, so are we. Indeed, we are ever-evolving always improving unfinished beings. Isn't it splendid to know we can always learn, grow, change, and become who we are meant to be at any given moment in time? We can always do better and be better. This I have learned over two decades of trying to do right for myself with the weight loss surgery I promised I would use wisely. It takes so much work, but there is always, always hope and promise. We never lose that potential.

What are you worth? As I spend my days meeting people in our ever-growing (yet shrinking) weight loss surgery world I frequently meet those who have lost a feeling of personal worth. Perhaps obesity caused feelings of worthlessness. Maybe unkindness or abuse from others had scarred us. Life experiences have a way of bringing us down and there was a time I believed myself worthless. Worthlessness, defined as devoid of worth, use or value, is a terrible place to be.

But I submit that all individuals are born of worth and value; all humans are born priceless. Our experiences, our achievements, our mistakes do not change our worth: they build our character. They define our personality. We have wellness and we have illness, but we never lose our worth.

Consider two $100 bills: one is old and worn, bent, crinkled and tired. The other pristine with nary a blemish or scar. Which piece of currency is worth more? They are both worth the same: $100. Experience and wear cannot diminish the value of the worn $100 bill: it tells a story. Perhaps the bill bought a single mother a basket of groceries. Maybe a grandmother sent it lovingly in a card to a grandchild. Maybe a drug addict traded the bill for a fix. Maybe a dad gave it to his son for his first date and said, "Treat the young lady nicely."

Visible wear and tear speaks the story. As people battling morbid obesity our bodies show wear and tear. Our emotions and our hearts may be blemished and bruised, but our worth is in place. We only need to recognize it.

Society would have us believe we are people of lesser value, a people of sloth and gluttony. There are those who would diminish our value as we take-up space in a world of pretty people. But I beg to say that those people are equally blemished and have the scars of wear and tear just as profound as they presume ours to be. If a person has been engaged in living life, then without exception they have wear and tear. The wear and tear tell a story, but it doesn't change one's worth.

And let's not forget the pristine $100 bill. What potential it holds! Perhaps it will travel through a Salvation Army bucket or pay the bill to heat a cold winter home or take a child to Disneyland or buy the elderly a much-needed prescription. I hope it passes hands many times never losing its worth.

> *"People change and forget to tell each other."*
> *--Lilliam Hellman*

Become Your Own Real. Not long ago I consulted with a young woman who is considering having a surgical weight loss procedure to take control of her obesity and her health. She is certain this is the right option for her. Her husband is concerned that weight loss surgery will change the person she is and that it will negatively affect their relationship. She promised him, *"I will always be the same person, and weight loss surgery will not change me."*

Do you remember making that promise to someone whose relationship was important to you? I certainly made that naive promise and I believed it was the truth. But weight loss surgery did change me, some for the good, some for the bad: all part of my personal evolution as a living breathing ever-learning human being.

And those changes affected every relationship in my life. After losing weight I was not available to eat with my former food-buddies because my free time was more happily enjoyed in the activities of living. Soon I felt isolated and rejected in many relationships. Later I learned that my friends of many years felt betrayed and abandoned when I no longer wanted to do the things we had always done together. Much of our socializing was sedentary eating and drinking and my choice for weight loss surgery trumped the choice to continue that activity. It was a harsh blow to me when a close friend said, "I do not like who you are now," at a time when I felt like I was the best me I had ever been.

One reason change is so profound with weight loss surgery is that physical change occurs rapidly in the grand scheme of a lifetime. Consider that in a year a person with weight loss surgery is quite capable of becoming physically half the person they once were.

Another reason for our dramatic change is the tendency for obese men and women to withdraw, to choke down their true person and disappear inside, hiding from a world where we are judged so harshly. In 1943 Sylvia Ashton-Warner wrote, "How much of my true self I camouflage and choke, denying the fullness of me. How I've toned myself down, diluted myself to maintain approval." Can you relate? Yet when we lose weight, we seemingly gain the courage to emerge from this prism that has misrepresented us for many years and find our true self.

And that is what it ultimately comes down to: being true to our self and finding inner peace. We can divorce a spouse or break a friendship, but we cannot divorce our self. Nathaniel Branden in "The Psychology of Self-

Esteem" writes, "When we bury feelings, we also bury ourselves. It means we exist in a state of alienation. We rarely know it, but we are lonely for ourselves."

Do you remember that wonderful childhood storybook "*The Velveteen Rabbit*" by Margery Williams? On Christmas morning the Boy, as he is called, finds a Velveteen Rabbit and plays with it until other toys distract him and the rabbit is set aside. Soon the Velveteen Rabbit was just another toy in the nursery, but he befriends the Skin Horse. As the Velveteen Rabbit expresses his wishes to be real the Skin Horse patiently explains, "Real isn't how you are made. It's a thing that happens to you. When a child loves you for a long, long time, not just to play with, but really loves you, then you become real."

Our task is to let our inner child really, really love our true emerging and ever-changing wonderful self. "As you learn to acknowledge, accept, and appreciate what it is that makes you different from all the other men and women in the world, the process begins," writes Sarah Ban Breathnach in Simple Abundance. She continues, "As you learn to trust the wisdom of your heart and summon up the courage to make creative choices based on what you know is right for you, process becomes progress."

It is Okay that we change with weight loss surgery. And it is inevitable. While those around us may reject that change it is most important to be forever true to ourselves. Do not choke down your true person and hide inside just because your relationships are challenged. Love yourself like the Boy loved his Velveteen Rabbit and become your own "Real".

Before you go. Thank you so much for staying with me for this conversation. I want to share one more thing before you go (hopefully to the next chapters). This is an essential part of what Day 6 is all about and I say this from my heart: You are worthy of your own care giving. Please, allow me to say it again.

You are worthy of your own care giving. We are notorious for being stellar caregivers. You may be a nurse, a social worker, a teacher, a mom, a dad, a daughter, a son, a husband, a wife, a friend, a church member or a neighbor. Any of the above, I don't know. But what I do know is that for most of your life you have put the needs of others above yourself. You say yes more than you say no. You may go without dinner, but a sick and infirm elderly neighbor will not. You may cancel your medical appointment but not your child's. You will commiserate with a heartbroken coworker without asking for a shoulder to cry on over your own heartbreak. This I know about you.

You are worthy of your own care giving. You have extraordinary nurturing skills, but when it comes to nurturing yourself neglect often trumps kindness. I know. More days than not I am my last priority. So here together, you and I in conversation, let's enter a treaty to become our own caregiver.

Please do not panic. I am not asking for elaborate efforts or expenses such as a Caribbean spa cruise or two-hours of daily meditation although such luxuries would be nice. I suggest that you and I, together, approach a few things differently so that we may take better care of ourselves and we do not neglect our health or weight loss surgery. Little things genuinely improve our quality of living when applied thoughtfully.

The first little thing I ask you to try is this: stop beating yourself up for what you feel are shortcomings. This is not breaking news. But here is how I propose you do this: As we have been sharing this conversation, I have imagined you and I sharing tea on my comfy sofa. Now imagine that I confide in you the things I find self-loathing about myself. I really dump it on you, and it isn't pretty. You listen and let me give myself a 12-round beating. The same kind of beating our inner voices often deliver. After listening to me, your friend, what would you say to me? What advice and wisdom would you share to comfort me? What care giving would you provide me so that I could recover from the beating?

The next time your inner voice begins taking licks at your heart and soul, interrupt! Call a timeout, because that is probably what you did while you were listening to me. And become the caregiver to yourself that you were to me. You are worthy to be your own caregiver.

Kindness: Above all else, be kind to yourself, our ongoing theme. Express gratitude for your weight loss tool and for your personal empowerment. Celebrate doing the best you could to find a middle ground to respect yourself and your traditions. In any given week you will eat 21 meals. That means there are 21 meal opportunities to get it your plate right. Consider how powerful that makes you. Should one meal go astray you have 20 more opportunities to improve. Be kind to yourself and use a blown meal as an opportunity for acceptance and moving forward to nourish your body well.

Be the Guest. As nurturing people, we are known for our hospitality. Hospitality is the cordial reception of a guest, which is often considered invigorating or stimulating. Treat yourself as you would a guest. Think of a time when you were warmly welcomed as a guest and how that affable welcome elevated your mood. In that same manner, treat yourself as you would a cherished guest. My good friend and our inspiring Neighbor, Kim, is a single lady of refined elegance. Even if her companion is not with her for the evening meal at home she sets the table with lovely dishes, linens, and candles. She lowers the lights and plays soft music. Kim has a knack for making a plain pot of soup look five star. In so doing, she elevates her mood. She is a cherished guest at her own table.

Ask for help. When we enjoyed the online Neighborhood I received letters from Neighbors who had gone missing from the community. They start, "Sorry I haven't been around the community, I've been struggling lately." It is an odd thing that at times when we most need help we retreat. Let me assure you, there is always someone doing well who has strength to spare.

When you are struggling don't retreat. Ask for help. In the karma of life your turn will come around to give back in another's time of need.

Seek Support. In talking to WLS groups I often quote the narrative from the beautiful movie March of the Penguins. Morgan Freeman opens the film saying, "Technically the emperor penguin is a bird although one who makes his home in the sea. He will leave the comfort of his own home and embark on a remarkable journey. He will travel great distance and though he is a bird he will not fly. Though he lives in the sea he will not swim. Mostly he will walk. But he will not walk alone." It is impossible not to draw a parallel with the weight loss surgery community because we, by having surgery, are doing something that is counterintuitive to everything we know. We are making a remarkable journey against the odds of our genetic nature and we are traveling in a harsh and unforgiving environment.

But like the penguin, we need not walk alone. As the story unfolds, we learn survival is in the group huddle: a united mass and cooperative team. The narrator describes, "As winter descends the tribe's only defense against the freezing cold is the group itself. The huddled animals form a single moving mass; one designed for the sole purpose of sustaining warmth."

Like the penguins we, the WLS Tribe, must sustain warmth and protection from our own harsh environment by becoming a huddled mass designed to sustain life and enable not just survival but success as we fight for our health in this unforgiving environment. So often I receive letters from people who tell me they feel alone in their journey after WLS. At one time I, too, felt alone without friend or traveling companion. Like the penguin, traveling this journey alone is risky; we need our huddled mass to survive. Of the solo penguin the narrator says, "The lone penguin has no chance against winter's cold. He will simply fade away absolved by the great whiteness around him."

We cannot let our fellow weight loss surgery neighbors simply fade away. We must gather the tribe together in a life-giving mass. Ours, like the penguins, can be a story of love, perseverance, commitment, survival, and triumph in the harshest conditions of nature and environment.

You know what? We just ate ourselves silly!

--The Mean Grandma

Be Silly. I think that sometimes in the intensity of trying to do all the right things with this weight loss surgery we take ourselves too seriously. We forget that laughter is the best medicine. My grandmother Rhoda, who would have loved sharing tea with us today, taught me about the healing power of silliness.

It was the summer of my twelfth year on a small farm in the middle of no-where Idaho that Grandma Rhoda taught me to eat myself silly. Far away from home and friends, the summer of 1978 was pretty much about Grandma Rhoda and me. Quietly I feared the family matriarch. She was a stern no-nonsense taskmaster. Secretly, us kids, we called her, "The Mean Grandma." I am certain I cried as my family waved goodbye from the car exiting the drive. Six weeks was a long time to spend with "The Mean Grandma."

Grandma Rhoda saw my tears and whisked me inside the immaculately clean farmhouse. Aqua green melamine dishes were stacked in the dish drying rack and the big black clock, all the way from Puerto Rico, ticked loudly through the sparse uncluttered house. My eyes must have been as big as moons as I watched Grandma Rhoda and her generous girth bend to pull an old aluminum cake pan from a low cupboard. With military efficiency she filled the pan with jars of homemade pickles, saltine crackers and slices of cheese. To that she added a bowl of ruby red raspberries she harvested at dawn from her own patch. With a satisfied nod she sternly directed, "Come with me."

The pebbled drive was warm under my bare feet as I followed The Mean Grandma past the open-port garage; along the riot-of-color flowerbed. I watched my big Swedish grandmother plop on the grass under the shade of an old, fruit-heavy, apple tree. She motioned me to her side. I sat quietly and watched. Grandma Rhoda placed a slice of cheese a top a saltine and added a slice of sweet pickle to that. She made a second, a third and a fourth. Then she served me and enjoyed a cracker stack herself. We had a second cracker each, munching in silence. Then she sat the bowl of ruby red raspberries between us and said, "Try one: it is like eating sunshine." The curiously soft, furry berry melted in my mouth in a burst of sweet-red ripeness. I was hooked. Together, she and I, we sat; eating one-by-one, little bites of sunshine.

Then it happened. The Mean Grandma giggled. A big loud happy belly-rolling giggle; and the giggle got bigger and bigger and bigger. My fright turned to laughter and I started to giggle too! She stuck out her tongue to show me the raspberry stains and I did the same back to her. And we giggled. She pulled a hanky from the sleeve of her housedress and used it to wipe the tears from her eyes. And then we giggled some more.

Pretty soon we were giggled out and Grandma Rhoda said to me, "You know what? We just ate ourselves silly!"

Those six weeks went by quickly. Many afternoons Grandma Rhoda and I could be found under that old apple tree eating ourselves silly. And so it went, in the summer of my twelfth year, that I learned from The Mean Grandma the most precious of lessons: simple food, cool shade, quiet companionship, warm sun kissed raspberries, and eating myself silly. Grandma Rhoda told me often, "It doesn't get better than this."

When it all becomes too much, step back, and entertain thoughts of your own silliness or perhaps invent some new silliness. The memory of silliness my grandmother gave me is etched upon my heart forever. I hope I can make a silliness memory along to someone I cherish. The adage is true that laughter is the best medicine and it is one of the simplest things to do.

You would have liked Grandma Rhoda and she would have liked and understood you. She struggled with her weight all her life. And right now she would offer you more tea with a wedge of lemon.

Thank you for being my guest. I have so much enjoyed your company and the opportunity you have given me to share some of my observations along the path of weight loss surgery this last ten years. As you travel through these pages my continuing message is that I believe in you. I see the hurt and the hope in your eyes and in your heart. I understand the challenges you face, but I know there are magnificent triumphs as well. My heart is yours, as are my prayers. I believe in you.

CHAPTER 2: FOUR RULES REVIEWED

S peaking in generalities, the "Four Rules" are the standard instructions provided most patients who undergo a surgical procedure for weight loss. The Four Rules are: Protein First; Lots of Water; No Snacking and Daily Exercise. These are the rules I was taught before surgery and was asked to recite after surgery before being released from my surgeon's care. These are the rules, two decades later, by which I live. These are the rules that work for me.

I say, speaking in generalities because over the years with different procedures and different programs there have been different twists to the rules. You may have been instructed differently and something different may be working for you. I respect that and I do not seek to convert anyone to these rules, particularly if what you have been instructed is working for you. My goal here is to share what I was taught, the same of, which remains the standard prescribed post-WLS curriculum, and offer hints for how I keep it fresh and working for me. At all times I strongly encourage you to follow the basics prescribed by your surgeon and bariatric center based on the procedure you had. They know what is best for you.

RULE #1 - PROTEIN FIRST

The first rule for living after Weight Loss Surgery is Protein First. That means eating protein for three daily meals, and protein must be 50 percent of total food intake. Current recommendations based on a 1,200-calorie diet are for 60-105g protein per day. Animal products are the most nutrient rich source of protein and include fish, shellfish, poultry and meat. Dairy protein, including eggs, is another excellent source of protein. On average, one ounce of animal or dairy protein contains 6-7 grams of protein. Nuts and legumes are a fair source of protein but significantly higher in fat than carefully selected lean animal protein. Also, due to their high fiber content, they may be more difficult for some gastric surgery patients to digest.

Protein intake is so important it deserves its own book. Get a copy of "Protein First: Understanding & Living the First Rule of Weight Loss Surgery" by Kaye Bailey available in paperback and digital formats at your favorite online book retailer. This little book is packed with information you need to understand and live the Protein First rule. When you understand and live *Protein First* after bariatric surgery you will achieve optimal weight loss and maintain a healthy weight for the remainder of your well-lived days.

A high protein diet for weight loss is not a new discovery. In fact, as early as 1825 a French lawyer and food lover Jean-Anthelme Brillat-Savarin published an essay: "Preventative or Curative Treatment of Obesity." Brillat-Savarin writes, *"Now, an antifat diet is based on the commonest and most active cause of obesity, since, as it has already been clearly shown, it is only because of grains and starches that fatty congestion can occur, as much in a man as in the animals; this effect plays a large part in the commerce of fattened beasts for our markets, and it can be deduced, as an exact consequence, that a more or less rigid abstinence from everything that is starchy or floury will lead to the lessening of weight."* Brillat-Savarin made his conclusions nearly 185 years ago. Today, here in cattle country where I live, we still send our beef to market fattened on grain and we still lose weight on a diet restricted of grains and starches. He was not so far off the mark.

The difference is that now we understand how and why a high protein diet works. First, of the four food elements (carbohydrate, fat, protein, and

36

alcohol) protein has the highest thermic effect at 20-30%. That means the energy expended during digestion and absorption of protein is 20-30% more than the energy (caloric) content of the food. It takes more energy (calories) to digest and absorb protein than the energy (calories) the protein contains. In processing protein your body must tap into stored energy resources (fat) to get the job done. No wonder a high protein diet supports fat (weight) loss.

Even after healthy body weight is achieved a high protein diet is necessary to maintain weight and avoid weight regain. High quality protein is essential to our well-being because it contains the compounds composed of carbon, hydrogen, oxygen, and nitrogen atoms that are arranged into amino acids linked in a chain that build strong muscles and bones, cause blood to clot, give us sight, and lend structure to all body parts. Amino acids are essential to our immune, cardiovascular and respiratory systems. Amino acids give us life. The Protein First rule is for life. Most centers recommend patients consume 60 to 105g protein a day for the rest of their life following gastric surgery for weight loss.

There are times when it will feel much more comfortable to eat carbohydrates, particularly soft processed carbohydrates, instead of lean protein. However, in order to maintain a healthy weight and avoid weight gain we must be ever vigilant in following the Protein First rule always.

RULE #2 - LOTS OF WATER

Dieters are often told drink water. Drink a minimum of 64 ounces a day: eight 8-ounce glasses a day. Gastric-bypass patients don't have a choice: they must drink lots water. Other beverages including coffee, tea, milk, soft drinks, and alcohol are discouraged. Water is the essential fluid for living. Water is one of the most important nutrients the body requires to stay healthy, vibrant and energetic.

The human body is a magnificent vessel full of water. The brain is more than 75 percent water and 80 percent of blood is water. In fact, water plays a critical role in every system of the human body. Water regulates body temperature, removes wastes, carries nutrients and oxygen to the cells, cushions the joints, prevents constipation, flushes toxins from the kidneys and liver and dissolves vitamins, minerals and other nutrients for the body's use.

The body will panic if actual water intake is significantly less than required. Blood cannot flow, waste processes are disrupted, and the electrolytes become imbalanced. Proper hydration prevents inflammation, promotes osmosis and moistens lung surfaces for gas diffusion. It helps the body regulate temperature, irrigate the cells and organs and promotes all functions of elimination. Theory suggests by drinking plenty of water many people could resolve inflammation and elimination problems that result from insufficient water intake. Adequate water facilitates weight loss.

In addition, the mind often confuses the body's cry for hydration as a cry for food. When hunger pangs strike it is wise to first have a glass of water and wait to see if feelings of hunger decrease before reaching for food. We can save many calories when we treat our thirst with water and save our calories for treating true hunger.

"Can I count my coffee as my water?" I get this question frequently. It frustrates me. Now, I enjoy a delicious cup of coffee in the morning just as much as the next person. But honestly, especially during the phase of weight loss, do we really need to ask one more thing of our body? All it wants is some water to flush away the toxins and fat we have been storing for years. The cellular process is working around the clock to do this for us. Don't we owe it to our body to give it a good flushing with water throughout the day? Enjoy your coffee but not in the place of water

In recent years several quality products have come to market that enhance water and make it palatable for non-water drinkers. One of my favorites is

Kellog's™ Special K2O Protein Water Mix. It is a sweet flavored powder that when mixed with water adds 5 grams of protein to 20 fluid ounces of water. At full strength this is a bit sweet for my taste but over ice it is a refreshing change for me. And who doesn't mind getting in a little extra protein here and there? You will find this near the vitamins and dietary supplements in your supermarket and discount stores.

RULE #3 - NO SNACKING

Without a doubt, the "No Snacking" rule is the most divisive in the weight loss surgery community. In fact, I've received more angry letters on this topic than any other of the Four Rules. One school of thought is that snacking is absolutely forbidden. The other school swears that three meals plus two snacks a day are essential for the nutritional survival of the weight loss surgery patient.

I am not a doctor and I am not a nutritionist. But I work on the front lines with weight loss surgery patients every day, patients who are many years out from surgery; patients who have lost touch with their bariatric centers. What I do know for certain is this: patients who snack and who are not engaged in extreme athletics gain weight. There is a fine line between snacking intelligently and grazing and few, if any, of us have the self-control to toe the line. In my experience and in my opinion, there is no reason for the average person post-WLS to ever engage in snacking. If we follow the DAY 6 DIET we will not be hungry in the 4-6 hours between planned meals; there will not be a blood glucose emergency and there will not be a physiological need to snack.

Taking a hardline against snacking is an unpopular position. But I have spent the last six years working with my fellow weight loss surgery patients and in every case of weight regain snacking has been involved. And in most cases the initial instructions from the bariatric center were for the patient to eat every 3 to 4 hours and somewhere along the third-year things went wrong. Snacking on protein bars or nuts became grazing on pretzels and crackers washed down with soda, coffee or tea. Slider foods overruled sensibility.

No Snacking. It is the rule that works.

Now, I'm obligated to tell you to follow the specific instructions given you by your bariatric center. If they advised three meals a day and two snacks a day that's fine: please do not feel I'm criticizing. But please, go get your original notes and instructions. Review the list of approved snacks. Copy that list and post it on your refrigerator to keep your memory refreshed. The snacks your center permitted during the phase of weight loss are the only snacks you are allowed for the rest of your life if you want to maintain your weight loss.

I personally feel the "NO Snacking" rule is a tremendous relief. For several years of my adult life, prior to surgery, I had a 40-minute commute to and from work each day. My morbidly obese irrational thinking had me convinced that I could not last that commute without a large soda and giant cookie: both morning and night. Looking back that was about 1,200 calories of snacking I was taking each day just to "survive" my commute. Twelve hundred calories is equal to our prescribed daily caloric allowance after surgery! How was it again, that I became morbidly obese? Hmmm. My car was always full of crumbs and the back seat littered with empty cups and cookie wrappers, not to mention the expense of my snacking habit. What a relief when "No Snacking" took that burden from me.

One reason we are prone to break the "No Snacking" rule is because traditional snack foods are ever present in our society and they tend to set more comfortably in our stomach pouch than protein dense food. Have you found yourself able to eat an endless bag of crackers or chips yet struggle to get a few bites of roast chicken down? The crackers are soft and when consumed with liquid create slurry that never compacts in the pouch the way protein does. The cracker slurry slides right through in a steady stream: slider food (more on this in Part II: DAY 6 DIET Basics). Solid protein, on the other hand, settles in the pouch like an unwelcome second cousin on your sofa and lingers just a little too long. So naturally we prefer to eat something that gives us comfort, not discomfort.

But the fact is, the pouch when it is used correctly, is supposed to be a little bit uncomfortable. The discomfort is the signal to stop eating. When we are snacking on slider food we do not get that signal and we do not stop eating.

Snacking Hazard: Slider Foods : Did you know that regardless of bariatric procedure, patients who experience weight regain after weight loss with surgery cite eating slider foods as the primary cause of weight regain?

To the weight loss surgery patient slider foods are the bane of good intentions often causing dumping syndrome, weight loss plateaus, and eventually weight gain. Slider foods are soft simple processed carbohydrates of little or no nutritional value that slide right through the surgical stomach pouch without providing nutrition or satiation.

Most Commonly Consumed Slider Foods after WLS: Pretzels, crackers (saltines, graham, Ritz®, Wheat Thins, etc.) filled cracker snacks such as Ritz Bits®, popcorn, cheese snacks (Cheetos®) or cheese crackers, tortilla chips with salsa, potato chips, sugar-free cookies, sweets, cakes, and candy. You will notice these are the same foods to contribute to dumping syndrome as described later in this chapter.

Why is it that we turn to these foods following surgery? We know that they contribute to obesity because they were likely a part of our diet prior to surgery. Common sense tells us that if food contributed to our obesity before surgery it will surely cause weight gain after surgery. We promised our surgeon to follow the dietary rules after surgery, yet somehow that grit determination wanes and little by little we find our old comfort food snacks back in hand. Reverting to the old dietary habits happens quite subtly and before we know it the scale is going in the wrong direction. "Now what?" we ask ourselves and then incite internal blame for yet another failed weight management effort. But before we jump on the self-loathing wagon let's consider the mechanical reasons that so many of us turn to slider foods even though we know they don't support our health and weight management goals.

Pouch Discomfort: the pouch makes us do it. From the 5DPT Owner's manual, "The very nature of the surgical gastric pouch is to cause feelings of tightness or restriction when one has eaten enough food. However, when soft simple carbohydrates are eaten this tightness or restriction does not result and one can continue to eat, unmeasured amounts of food without ever feeling uncomfortable. Many patients unknowingly turn to slider foods for this reason. They do not like the discomfort that results when the pouch is tightens from eating a measured portion of lean animal or dairy protein, and it is more comfortable to eat the soft slider foods." I've spoken with thousands of WLS patients over the years and it is strikingly common to hear saltine crackers implicated as the first food encountered leading to slider food snacking. It happens innocently enough when discomfort is experienced when eating animal protein.

This discomfort can be pouch tightness, nausea, repulsion to taste or texture, and physical fatigue immediately following the meal. When we are following the liquid restrictions (no beverage 30 minutes before or after a meal, no beverage with the meal) a high-protein meal can feel heavy and pouch tightness results quickly, possibly before we realize it and stop eating. I have occasional spells of extreme frustration brought on by the discomfort of the pouch when I'm following the rules. Sometimes eating Protein First feels like a punishment and a high price to pay to keep my weight in check.

Memory lapse. Remarkably, the most common time for us to return to slider snacks is after we have lost a goodly amount of weight and are feeling healthy and well. Is it possible that we forget just how bad obesity made us feel? On page 16 of the 5DPT Owner's Manual 2nd Edition I write, "It is a funny thing, the way the mind works. The healthier we become the less we remember how truly sick we were before surgery and before weight loss. Like the memory of pain reported following childbirth, findings indicate that the more positive our experience is with weight loss, the less vividly we recall the pain (physical and emotional) of obesity prior to weight loss. This suggests that when we fall off the wagon of dietary compliance it is not so much about a moral breakdown or relenting to environmental pressure (think food pushers), but perhaps we simply don't remember how bad obesity felt."

Weight regain attributed to consumption of slider foods brings with it a bag of negative emotions and self-blame. Confessions of "being bad" are common when patients are eating soft non-nutritional carbohydrates. Adjectives describe these foods as bad, evil, sinful, decadent, self-indulgent, wicked, etc. You get the idea. We call ourselves bad, weak, powerless, pathetic, sloppy, stressed, and anything else morally incriminating as we vow to be good tomorrow. But here's the thing: food cannot be bad or evil or sinful because food is inert – without energy or motivation - and has no morals. Food is sustenance. It can taste good or bad, but it cannot be good or bad. This is an important concept because once we release food of moral attributes, we can more rationally deal with our food choices taking guilt and self-loathing out of the equation. We live in a world where we face food choices at every turn. Sometimes we chose healthy sustenance and other times our choice is nutritionally deficient.

The selection of a nutritionally void slider food is not a catastrophe brought on by moral weakness: it is just a choice.

Another choice awaits at the next meal that is completely independent of the previous choice. This is an opportunity to support our health goals and desires by selecting something nutritionally abundant that complies with our Protein First WLS diet.

Rule #4 - Daily Exercise

The final rule, the one many weight loss surgery post-ops despise the most: patients must exercise every day.

Nothing is more disappointing than hearing a gastric bypass patient brag that they did not have to exercise to lose weight. It is true; patients will lose weight without lifting a finger. But patients who do not use the time of rapid weight loss to incorporate exercise into their lifestyle are doing themselves a grave disservice.

Obesity cripples the body. Bone tissues are compromised, joints are swollen, the vascular system is inadequate and the skeleton overburdened. As weight is lost, the burden on the bones, joints and vascular system is decreased. However, the body is a magnificent machine. Given proper nutrition and physical motion it will rebuild its broken framework. The systems can become strong and vital.

The most effective way to heal the body from the ravages of obesity is to exercise. Exercise means moving the body: walking, stretching, bending, inhaling and exhaling. Exercise is the most effective, most enjoyable, most beneficial gift one can bestow upon oneself in the recovery from life threatening, crippling morbid obesity. People who successfully maintain their weight exercise daily.

Let me tell you about the *Training Room Tyrant* who in a single day broke my spirit in what I believed was a genuine attempt at physical fitness during my sophomore year of college. Two fatty friends and I joined an early morning weight training class so we could become powerful and strong. He, our instructor, was lean, fit, and fine to look at. And he was a fat bigot. He barked orders like a prison warden and belittled us for being fat girls. Certainly, we were fat by choice, out-of-control gluttons. But fat girls like to please; we yearned to be accepted in an unforgiving world. Without complaint we lifted, tugged and pulled on weights that were much too heavy too many times on this our first day of class. The more we tried to please the Tyrant the more he pushed.

We spent the next four days in hell. Our entire muscular systems were broken and ripped: we suffered physical injury and emotional shame. Several days later our muscles healed, but our spirits remained shattered. We felt like unworthy little pigs living in a thin man's world. So, we did what fat girls do; we ate ourselves better, drowning our sorrows in tubs of ice cream. We never went back to class. And even though I spent but 40 minutes under his command I never forgot the Training Room Tyrant.

Years later and a few weeks after bariatric surgery I stepped on my treadmill and I spent ten minutes walking laboriously. With every slow steady step I took I cursed the Tyrant and I vowed to avenge the shame and humiliation he had wrought upon my compatriots and me. And the next day I walked and I was mad as hell at the Tyrant. And I saw all the others who had belittled me throughout my life and I avenged myself with every step. Every day I walked madder and faster and further fueled by my anger. "I'll-show-them, I'll-show-them" sang the cadence of my step.

Then one day I noticed how great it felt to fill my lungs with air, and exhale effortlessly. My legs were strong, my heart beat steady and I was becoming a fit person. My body became strong and I pulled myself tall with confident posture. I loved swinging my arms to every step. I put music on the stereo and turned it up loud! I walked for me – for the pure joy of motion. And the anger slipped away. When I let this anger go it was replaced with positive thoughts and the countless wounds inflicted upon my spirit over the years began to heal. I had triumphed! At last the victory was mine.

Exercise need not be fancy or formal. It can be a walk around the block or a romp on the floor with the children, the grandchildren or the puppy and the pets. It can be lifting the bag of groceries from the car or taking a flight of stairs instead of the elevator. It just simply means moving these beautiful precious bodies of ours. If you can, take an extra step. Lift an extra bit of weight. Reach a little further. Move a little faster. Every motion helps, every movement makes forward progress toward better health. And you are worth it.

The most common "Obstacles" I hear from people who elect not to use exercise with their WLS tool are: lack of time; too busy to exercise; too embarrassed to exercise in public; waiting until after losing the weight; can't afford gym membership; or simply do not like exercise. These are excuses, not obstacles.

Again, I will take an unpopular stand here and state that if we went to the trouble, risk and cost to have weight loss surgery we have no room for excuses. Exercise is non-negotiable. Now, I am not saying you must run a marathon or lift your body weight on the bench press. I'm saying we must take an extra step; we must stretch and flex, and we must lift a little more. We must do just a little bit more each day to build a stronger body. Babies do not go from the bumper chair to running in a day; neither should we. By the same token, we cannot stay sedentary and expect to achieve a healthful recovery from morbid obesity.

THE DISCOMFORT FACTOR OF THE FOUR RULES

The intended outcome of restrictive gastric surgery is to cause tolerable discomfort –*think post-Thanksgiving dinner*-- after eating a small portion of food. When we follow the rules eating lean protein with limited complex carbohydrates without liquids, the dense food matter, chyme, fills our stomach pouch quickly and densely with a small amount of food volume. The density causes a tight feeling that is uncomfortable. The desired result is that we stop eating when we feel discomfort or fullness.

In many cases the discomfort of a full pouch is accompanied by feelings of nausea. If we ignore the discomfort and continue to eat it is likely we will vomit. This is how the pouch is intended to work: the discomfort signals us to stop eating or we reject the food by vomiting.

If we understand this discomfort as a desired result of eating enough, we learn to stop short of the discomfort and nausea and over time appreciate the one-bite-under sense of satiation.

Unfortunately, though no fault of our own, we are disposed to find a more comfortable way of eating which ultimately leads us off course. In weight loss surgery street talk we call it "eating around the pouch". Yet I dare say finding a more comfortable way of eating is more adaptation than deliberate disobedience to the new rules we have been taught.

It begins with the reintroduction of liquids or moisture with meals. We do not do this as a flagrant in-your-face show of rebellion; we are simply seeking a way to make eating more comfortable. Remember, we have spent our entire life seeking comfort in eating. I can recall during the first year following surgery preferring stewed chicken cacciatore to dry skillet chicken breasts because the moist preparation caused less discomfort for me. Braised and stewed protein preparations became my first choice over lean undressed proteins. This led way to the inclusion of sips with meals and a more comfortable relationship with my pouch following meals.

Like so many others, I learned to eat around my pouch eventually enjoying graham crackers and coffee: slider-food slurry. I was back in comfort food heaven. But as we know, comfort food heaven takes us to weight gain hell.

When we follow the weight loss surgery rules our body will feel discomfort when the pouch is full. This is the signal to stop eating. Practiced listening to this signal and monitoring how long it takes from plate to pouch to get there will eventually allow us to stop one-bite-short of discomfort. We will experience satiation and feel appreciation for our pouch.

Finding acceptance, respect and comfort for how the gastric pouch works is a challenge we will face for the rest of our lives. Our call to action is to make the pouch work when it is contrary to everything we have known up to the point of surgery. We must actively contrive a plan to work in concert with the pouch if we intend to go beyond the Four Rules and enjoy lifelong health and weight maintenance using our surgical tool.

DUMPING SYNDROME: RAPID GASTRIC EMPTYING

Dumping syndrome is a phenomenon, primarily reserved for Gastric Bypass Roux-en-Y patients which is characterized by unpleasant symptoms when the patient's blood sugar is adversely affected by simple sugars, simple carbohydrates, and fatty foods. When these foods are rapidly absorbed by the small intestine dumping syndrome may occur. Some Roux-en-Y patients never seem to experience dumping, others are surprised when some foods trigger an episode and others do not, and still there is always the surprise dumping event that occurs on food that has previously been enjoyed without incident. Let's take a deep dive into dumping syndrome and consider actions to prevent it. You will also find a recipe for Spinach-

Ginger soup that is made of healing ingredients and soothes a distressed tummy. Give it a try next time you have a grumpy pouch day.

In a gastric bypass Roux-en-Y the connection between the pouch and the small intestine is the cause of food intolerance we refer to as dumping or dumping syndrome. This intolerance is the direct result of food, usually higher in sugars and starches, entering directly into the small intestine having only mixed with saliva and not stomach acid. The symptoms of dumping syndrome may vary from person to person, but can include the following:

Sweating, rapid heartbeat, flushing skin, vomiting, shakiness, low blood pressure, dizziness, shortness of breath, diarrhea, fainting.

Although dumping syndrome may not seem desirable, it can be. For a gastric bypass patient, it can be a strong motivator to eat healthier, protein-dense foods and to avoid junk food. This has been referred to as forced behavior modification.

In Part II: Dietary Intelligence we provide first aid information for WLS patients who are experiencing a dumping incident.

FOODS THAT CAUSE DUMPING

As pre-op gastric bypass weight loss surgery patients we are taught to fear the mysterious dumping syndrome and instructed that avoiding sugar will prevent the occurrence of dumping syndrome. It comes as a surprise when after having a malabsorptive gastric surgery we experience symptoms that we think are dumping syndrome, yet sugar has not crossed our lips. Most information discussing dumping syndrome following weight loss surgery focuses on avoiding sugar and suggests that some patients "get" dumping syndrome while others do not get it, almost like it were an optional feature of the surgery. Other misinformation suggests that dumping syndrome goes away after time when patients adjust to surgery and eventually, they can tolerate sweets in increasing amounts.

Scant clinical research is published to help us understand dumping syndrome beyond personal experience. Combine the lack of reputable information with a plethora of urban legend about dumping syndrome and it is easy to understand the confusion.

Dumping syndrome, also called rapid gastric emptying, is defined by the National Digestive Diseases Information Clearinghouse (NDDIC) as, "a condition where ingested foods bypass the stomach too rapidly and enter the small intestine largely undigested. It happens when the upper end of the small intestine, the duodenum, expands too quickly due to the presence of hyperosmolar (substances with increased osmolarity) food from the stomach. "Early" dumping begins concurrently or immediately succeeding a meal." What that means to gastric bypass patients is that food particles are too quickly absorbed by the small intestine because they have gone directly there without the digestive benefits of an intact intestine. The food is literally "dumped" into the small intestine.

To manage this food the pancreas' releases excessive amounts of insulin into the bloodstream and the body experiences the symptoms of hypoglycemia. Symptoms may begin immediately or anytime within 3 hours of eating and may include nausea, vomiting, bloating, cramping, diarrhea, dizziness and fatigue. Symptoms do subside as insulin levels return to normal. Many patients experiencing dumping find comfort in lying down or sipping on fortified water or energy drinks served at room temperature.

Carbohydrates. The medical community generally agrees the treatment of dumping syndrome is through the avoidance of certain foods that cause it. People who have gastric dumping need to eat small meals that are high in lean protein, low in carbohydrates, avoid simple sugars, and should drink liquids between meals, not with meals. The following are three food groups that should be avoided in the treatment and prevention of dumping syndrome in gastric bypass patients:

- ○ *Simple Sugars*: cookies, cakes, candies, bakery items, ice cream, sweet dairy.
- ○ *Simple Carbohydrates:* chips, crackers, processed cereals, pasta with creamy milk sauces.
- ○ *High-Fat Carbohydrates*: French fries, deep fried food, fast food, grilled food with sweet barbecue sauce, cream-based soups and sauces.

A diet of carefully chosen lean protein with low glycemic fresh fruits and vegetables is effective in avoiding dumping syndrome. Ongoing research is beginning to implicate hyperinsulinemic hypoglycemia as the cause of rapid gastric emptying after weight loss surgery but for you and me on the front lines suffering from sweats and chills called dumping, what does that really mean right now? I suggest we become our own personal research scientists and develop a prudent dietary strategy based on current information and personal data that allows us to avoid dumping syndrome and lead a nutritionally balanced life.

Fried Foods. Anyone who is awake knows that fried food is not a healthy dietary choice. A high fat diet is believed to be a contributing cause of diabetes, heart disease, overweight and obesity. But Americans continue to load their plates with fried food because we have developed a taste for it and because food producers make products that taste good and are affordable.

Overweight people who have undergone bariatric weight loss surgery to control their weight are encouraged to follow a diet high in protein and low in fat and carbohydrate. This has been shown to effectively work with the weight loss surgery to reduce weight and control weight over long periods of time. Living in a world where high fat food is ever present, the surgical weight loss patient is often tempted to indulge in fried food often thinking that small amounts of fried food will not negatively affect their diet or health. However, eating fried food, even in small amounts, can have catastrophic consequences for gastric surgery patients.

In general, fried food is bad for us simply by the nature of its nutritional composition. Consider this: A 6-piece serving of fried chicken tenders contains 401 Calories; 16 grams Protein; 8 grams Fat; 57 grams Carbohydrate. The FDA calculates this at 3 1/2 starch/bread servings and 1 lean meat serving. It is easy to figure out how we have become "obese nation" when you consider many children are weaned from the bottle right to the fast food fried chicken pieces.

This nutritional data indicates the fried chicken tenders are a high fat carbohydrate. When a person who has undergone a malabsorptive gastric surgery such as gastric bypass eats high fat carbohydrates, they are at imminent risk of dumping syndrome. Gastric Dumping Syndrome, or rapid gastric emptying, is a condition where ingested foods bypass the stomach too rapidly and enter the small intestine largely undigested.

The syndrome is most often associated with malabsorptive gastric surgery, specifically gastric bypass surgery. Symptoms of dumping syndrome may manifest immediately after eating or within three hours of eating. Symptoms may include nausea, vomiting, bloating, cramping, diarrhea, dizziness and fatigue. Symptoms do subside as insulin levels return to normal. Many patients experiencing dumping find comfort in lying down or sipping on fortified water or energy drinks served at room temperature.

Not only is dumping syndrome physically uncomfortable it can be unpredictable and embarrassing. Many patients experience profuse sweating which can be embarrassing and difficult to explain to those unaware of the condition. At other times a patient may suffer from confusion and become disoriented which may appear to be intoxication or diabetic distress to someone unacquainted with the signs and symptoms of dumping syndrome.

The consequences of eating fried food after a gastric weight reduction surgery are twofold: immediate risk of dumping syndrome and long-term risk of weight gain and the diseases associated with a high-fat diet.

Gastric surgery patients, specifically gastric bypass patients, may prevent dumping syndrome by eating a diet of carefully chosen lean protein combined with low glycemic fresh fruits and vegetables. Patients are instructed to avoid simple sugars, simple carbohydrates and high-fat carbohydrates and to avoid drinking liquids with meals. At the onset weight loss surgery patients are instructed to eat a high protein diet following surgery.

SOOTHE STOMACH DISCOMFORT WITH SOUP

Talk to any gastric bypass, gastric banding or gastric sleeve patient and they will tell you occasional stomach discomfort is part of life after weight loss surgery. After bariatric surgery patients secrete fewer digestive enzymes which means the stomach has greater difficulty digesting food that has been inadequately chewed or is high in fat or fibrous carbohydrate. Poorly tolerated foods may quickly cause stomach or pouch discomfort. Many bariatric patients report finding relief in gentle homemade soup sipped slowly. Consider this recipe for spinach and ginger soup if you have experienced gastric pouch discomfort from eating poorly tolerated food.

SPINACH AND GINGER SOUP

This creamy green soup is delicately flavored with ginger and onion serves to soothe stomach discomfort and detoxify the body. The spinach is a natural immune system booster. The monounsaturated fat in the olive oil will help our bodies absorb the nutrients and minerals from the vegetables making this an ideal soup for pampering the gastric system.

Ingredients:
2 Tablespoons olive oil

1 medium onion, chopped
2 cloves garlic, finely chopped
2 teaspoons fresh ginger, finely chopped
5-6 cups young spinach leaves
4 cups vegetable stock
1 medium potato, diced
1 Tablespoon rice wine vinegar*
Salt and pepper, to taste
1 teaspoon sesame oil, optional

Directions: Heat the oil in a large 8-quart stockpot. Add the onion, garlic, and ginger and cook over low heat, stirring occasionally, for 3-4 minutes, or until vegetables are tender.

Set aside 4-6 small spinach leaves. Add the remaining leaves to the pan, stirring until the spinach is wilted. Add the stock and potatoes to the pan and bring to a boil. Reduce the heat, then cover the pan and let simmer for about 10 minutes.

Remove the pan from the heat and set aside to cool slightly. Pour the soup into a blender or food processor and process until completely smooth. Return the soup to the stockpot and add the rice wine vinegar. Adjust the seasoning to taste with salt and pepper. Heat until just about to boil.

Finely shred the reserved spinach leaves and sprinkle some over the top. Drizzle a few drops of sesame oil into the soup. Ladle into warmed soup bowls and sprinkle the remaining shredded spinach on each, then serve the soup at once.

Serves 4, 1 cup per serving. Per serving: 38 calories, 3 grams Protein; 2 grams Fat; 2 grams Carbohydrate.

*Rice Wine Vinegar: There are Japanese as well as Chinese rice vinegars, both made from fermented rice, and both slightly milder than most Western vinegars. Chinese rice vinegar comes in three types: white (clear or pale amber), used mainly in sweet-and-sour dishes; red, a popular accompaniment for boiled or steamed crab; and black, used mainly as a table condiment. The almost colorless Japanese rice vinegar is used in a variety of Japanese preparations, including sushi rice and salads. Rice vinegar can be found in Asian markets and some supermarkets.

WEIGHT LOSS RESISTANCE

Your body is fighting everything you do to lose weight. You and I, members of the weight loss surgery patient community, understand the endless battle against our own body when we take action to lose excess weight. We may not understand the metabolic science, but we know from experience that efforts to lose weight and keep it off are resisted by the body with the same hard-headed determination a rebellious teenager resists curfew.

We have excess body weight because a survival mechanism that stores excess body weight to prevent starvation is an over-achiever. The disease obesity is complicated by our evolution from hunter-gatherers for whom any weight loss was a threat to survival. To combat that threat the body evolved a physiological process to make it so weight could be easily and quickly regained.

"The body actually senses the weight loss as a threat to survival and begins to release hormones that lead to feelings of hunger to ensure a strong motivation to obtain as many calories as possible," says Los Angeles area bariatric surgeon Dr. Michael Feiz M.D., F.A.C.S . He explains that these biological processes may largely account for what is known as the "yo-yo" effect in which individuals manage to lose weight, only to quickly regain it.

I was among the many obesity sufferers who before weight loss surgery had managed to lose and regain significant weight several different times. What a head-trip this cycle is! The euphoria of weight loss followed by the shame and disappointment of weight regain. You too? I understand.

A 25 Million Year Process: Looking at the greater picture, the fight to los e weight is not singular against our own body: the fight is against 25 million years of human evolutionary history. "Humans are not self-made creations dietarily, but rather have an evolutionary history as anthropoid primates stretching back more than 25 million years," reports Katharine Milton in the American Journal of Clinical Nutrition. She continues, "This is a history that shaped their nutrient requirements and digestive physiology." We carry that history and the accompanying nutritional needs and metabolic physiology in our DNA.

In the personal struggle to manage obesity a nod to our ancestral evolution is in order. "It seems prudent for modern-day humans to remember their long evolutionary heritage as anthropoid primates and heed current recommendations," reports Milton. Such is easier said than done: the difficulty in treating obesity was formally recognized in 1958 when the Cornell Conference on Therapy reported, "Most obese patients will not remain in treatment, most will not lose significant poundage, most would regain it promptly."

Not much has changed in the 60 years since the Cornell Conference. Dr. Feiz explains that, while it is common knowledge that exercise and strict adherence to a balanced, low-calorie diet are surefire methods for weight loss, the difficulty of making sticking to low calorie diets over the long-term means that people with large amounts of excess weight to lose typically struggle both to lose it and, even more so, to keep it off. Dr. Feiz notes that one way in which bariatric surgery is effective is that it can address these physiological and hormonal factors that make dieting so difficult.

The Weight Loss Surgery Option: "For people with severe obesity and large amounts of excess weight to lose, weight loss surgery is the best medical intervention known to improve both the quality and length of their lives." Speaking specifically of the gastric sleeve procedure Dr. Feiz said, "This is a scientifically proven weight loss surgery technique that works in two ways. Firstly, the procedure removes a significant portion of the stomach, which makes its overall capacity much smaller. For the patient, this results in feeling satiated faster from smaller meals and servings.

Secondly, the procedure curbs the release of ghrelin, a hunger inducing hormone."

Surgery does not release patients from personal responsibility, but it does provide an eye-opening realization that obesity is a disease --a medical condition treated with major gastrointestinal surgery-- and sufferers must employ all means to fight responsibly against this ailment just as they would any other life-threatening condition. Dr. Feiz says, "Of course, the full benefits of the procedure are not attained unless the patient fulfills his or her commitment to eating significantly less overall. As part of treatment and recovery from obesity a program that includes a dietitian and counseling will guide the patients' changing relationship with food.

CHAPTER 3: 5 DAY POUCH TEST REVIEW

Before we begin the Day 6 Fundamentals let's review the basics of the 5 Day Pouch Test which will get you to Day 6. The 5 Day Pouch Test is a program I created, through much trial and error, to get back on track after experiencing a weight gain three years after surgery. When I contacted my bariatric center for help the counselor advised me to "get back to basics." Ashamed of my weight gain and feeling I had let my surgeon down, I was too embarrassed to ask, "What exactly does get back to basics mean?"

So, I pulled out my weight loss surgery binder and read every instruction sheet and piece of research I had collected. Then I made a plan that would mimic the early days and weeks following gastric bypass surgery. That was back to basics, wasn't it? It took several efforts and lots of adjusting before the 5 Day Pouch Test became the successful "back to basics" program it is today.

And what a powerful tool it has become in our world of weight loss surgery living. The 5 Day Pouch Test Owner's Manual has been shipped around the world and helped countless thousands who had lost confidence in their surgical weight loss tool. Never a day passes without hearing from someone who has rediscovered his or her pouch after following the 5 Day Pouch Test. It is empowering when we learn that our tool does work; it was our habits that caused us to gain weight or feel letdown by the surgery.

The most frequent question I hear after the 5 Day Pouch Test is "Now what?"

Hence you are holding this book. As a refresher the 5 Day Pouch Test is briefly summarized here. You may read the complete plan online at www.5daypouchtest.com. The 5 Day Pouch Test Owner's Manual by Kaye Bailey is available for purchase on that website. And be sure to click on the newsletter subscription button to receive the free email: 5 Day Pouch Test Bulletin. It is full of tips, recipes and inspiration. You will meet others, just like you, who want to do their best with weight loss surgery.

The 5 Day Pouch Test is a plan to determine if the surgical stomach pouch is working and return to that tight newbie feeling. It is effective with all gastric weight loss procedures. It is helpful in returning to the dietary basics we practiced after surgical weight loss. It is not difficult to follow and if you are in a stage of carbohydrate addiction it will help break the cycle.

The 5 Day Pouch Test is not a diet and the intent is not for the singular express purpose of losing weight, although many report weight loss at the end of five days. When speaking I reassuringly tell my audience the 5 Day Pouch Test is their WLS airbag. You don't ever want to use it, but you know it is there if you need it. The 5DPT is intended to arrest out-of-control eating and halt weight gain. It is intended to return us to the way of eating that worked for us immediately after surgery.

It is only five days. And in those five days we learn that our pouch is working; we take control of our eating behaviors and we remind ourselves why we had weight loss surgery in the first place.

Days 1 and 2 of the plan are *healing* days. You treat your pouch like a newborn with gentle liquids and soups. Pouch inflammation is reduced, and processed carbohydrate cravings subside. Mental focus is on listening to and respecting your body. Days 1 and 2 mimic the early days and weeks following bariatric surgery.

Day 3 introduces soft proteins like canned fish, fresh soft fish and eggs. This is the day we focus on tasting our food, chewing well and enjoying the goodness of lean-clean protein. We focus on portion control and the liquid restrictions. On this day we start to remember what a tight pouch feels like and we appreciate the feeling of fullness.

Day 4 brings us to firm proteins like ground meat (beef, turkey, lamb, or game) and shellfish, scallops, lobster, salmon or halibut steaks. This is the day we truly realize the power of the pouch and most people are happily surprised to learn their pouch is not broken or stretched back to a normal size stomach, which technically is not possible. The carbohydrate withdrawal is over, and energy levels are improving.

Day 5 finishes the test with solid proteins such as white meat poultry, beefsteak, and any of the firm proteins from Day 4. The liquid restrictions are now a habit and we have successfully removed the slider foods from our diet. We have energy for exercise and for the daily tasks of living. Most importantly, we know our weight loss surgery tool works and we now have the confidence to work the tool.

Day 6 is the way we will eat every day for the rest of our lives. Having successfully broken a carb-cycle, gained a feeling of control over the surgical gastric pouch, and possibly having lost a few pounds we are ready to embrace the DAY 6 DIET. This means focusing on protein dense meals, observing the liquid restrictions, and avoiding starches, particularly processed carbohydrates and slider foods. Three meals a day should be two-thirds protein, one-third healthy carbohydrate in the form of low-glycemic vegetables and fruits. Consumption of whole grains is not forbidden but should be limited to one serving a day.

SLIDER FOODS & LIQUID RESTRICTIONS

Two key points the 5 Day Pouch Test remind us of are the danger of slider foods and the importance of liquid restrictions. In most cases, after careful assessment, those who experience weight gain or stalls in weight loss realize slider foods and relaxed liquid restrictions are to blame. Slider foods and Liquid restrictions are discussed in detail in Part II: DAY 6 DIET Basics.

5 DAY POUCH TEST FAQ'S

Q: What does 'broken my pouch' mean?
A: In the early weeks and months following gastric surgery there is a distinct feeling of tightness in the small stomach pouch created by the surgery. Small meals of dense protein and void of starch quickly bring a full feeling to a new post-op patient. This tightness triggers satiation for the patient: a strong signal of fullness. Weight loss results because of the decreased caloric consumption affected by the small gastric pouch.

As patients get further out from surgery there is a tendency to experiment with the pouch, perhaps including liquids with meals or eating foods that exit the pouch quickly, commonly called slider foods. In the worst-case slider foods are consumed with liquid; an example is graham crackers and coffee. In this case the coffee and graham crackers create slurry in the pouch and slide right through the outlet to the intestine, thus never filling the pouch. Caught quite unaware patients ask, "Is my pouch broken?" They report their pouch does not feel the same tightness as it did early post-op when the pouch was new, and they were compliant with the prescribed way of eating. When patients do the 5 Day Pouch Test, they are surprised to feel the pouch again simply by returning to the way of eating that worked in the first place after surgery.

Q: What happens after the 5DPT?
A: Beginning on Day 6 after the 5DPT we slowly include complex carbohydrate vegetables and fruit in the diet at a ratio of two-thirds protein to one-third complex carbohydrate when measured by volume. We continue to follow the liquid restrictions and avoid slider foods and stay intently focused on the Four Rules. Now that we have recaptured that hell-bent determination that propelled us to have surgery in the first place we

use the momentum in our pursuit of a healthy lifestyle and weight management with bariatric surgery.

Q: I did the 5DPT and lost weight, but it didn't stick. Why?

A: The motivation for doing the 5DPT should always be to get back on track with the WLS dietary guidelines, not to lose weight. That means we take what we learn during the 5 days and apply it to our lifestyle on Day 6 and beyond. If we do the 5DPT simply to knock-off a few pounds and then go back to the very habits that lead to weight regain we will, naturally, regain the weight and then some. When we consented to weight loss surgery, we agreed that for the rest of our life we would follow certain dietary guidelines. If we have drifted from the original guidelines the 5DPT can get us back to basics. At that point we must follow the guidelines we agreed to if we wish to sustain weight loss and keep our obesity in remission. Use this as part of a bigger strategy: returning to the instructions you were provided by your surgical weight loss center and nutritionist. Go back to doing what worked for you when you were at your best and losing weight or maintaining weight.

Q: What if the 5DPT shows me my pouch is broken?

A: If you have given the 5DPT your best effort and you still feel like your pouch is not working in the way it was intended to work please see your bariatric surgeon. Several diagnostic tests are available to determine the state of your pouch. In some instances, a surgical revision may be necessary due to a pouch failure. Notice it is a pouch failure, not a personal failure when a revision is necessary. Revisions for gastric surgery are common and sadly some needing revisions are made to feel like moral failures when this is not at all the case. A revision is a medical procedure to correct a medical condition. Seek the care of a qualified bariatric team and do what is necessary to protect your health.

Q: How soon can I do the 5DPT again?

A: Always keep in mind that the 5 Day Pouch Test is to be used a vehicle to get back on track with your WLS basics. It should not be used as a fad diet to quickly knock off a few pounds. Include the 5DPT in your weight management when you do not feel in control of your eating or cravings, when you have strayed from the Four Rules and basic tenets that have worked in the past to help you lose weight, and when you simply need to get back to the basics of WLS. Do the 5DPT when you are in a place mentally to take charge of your health and commit to getting back on track. This gives you the best chance for success. The focus should always be on learning to use the tools that will keep us on track for the long-term.

Q: If it is a liquid diet, why are soups allowed?
A: The 5 Day Pouch Test calls for two days of protein rich liquids. Normally we think of ready-to-drink protein beverages or homemade concoctions using fruit, yogurt and protein powder. This is quite typical of the early post-op diet prescribed by many surgical weight loss centers. The 5DPT begins with two days of protein liquids in order to baby the pouch, much as we did immediately post-op. In addition, the liquids are useful in breaking a processed carbohydrate snacking habit or slider food addiction.

Ideally one would spend Days 1 and 2 drinking only protein drinks, clear broth, tea and water. However, depending on your eating habits leading into the 5DPT this can be quite drastic causing hunger, dizziness and frustration. As I developed this plan, I learned that more substantial soups made of animal protein, legumes, beans and low-glycemic vegetables work well to alleviate the discomfort of a liquid diet.

These satisfying soup recipes are made of ingredients low on the Glycemic Index: a measure of how your blood glucose levels are affected by food. That means they will stick with you without causing a rapid rise (and then drop) in blood glucose. These great comfort soups will help keep you feeling full longer, help you achieve and maintain a healthy weight, and provide you with more consistent energy throughout the day.

It is easy to confuse soup with slider foods since both are liquids that flow more rapidly through the stoma than solid protein. But the thing to remember is the soup recipes recommended are nutrient dense. Slider foods such as crackers or pretzels washed down with liquids have no nutritional value. In addition, the soup is taken in a measured portion of 1 cup per serving. Seldom, when in slider food carbohydrate addiction, do we measure our portion.

A final note, the soup recipes I provide on the 5DPT are less expensive than processed protein beverages and they are family friendly making the 5 Day Pouch Test more practical to incorporate into our busy lives. The soups are so good you will want to include them in your Day 6 menu as well.

Q: Can I have vegetables on the 5 Day Pouch Test?

A: I am pleased that so many people include vegetables and fruit as part of their healthy post-WLS diet. Often labeled "good carbs" vegetables are an important part of our nutritional plan. But I dare say that few people have become out-of-control in a carb cycle eating vegetables or fruit. It is the simple carbohydrates (processed food or starches) that cause a carb-dependency due to the chemical imbalance of blood glucose levels.

The high protein diet we were prescribed after surgery works to facilitate weight loss because protein requires significant energy to digest: our bodies use stored energy (fat) just to process it. Protein is loaded with amino acids that make our bodies strong and bring about healing. When people report weight loss with the 5 Day Pouch Test it is because they have pushed their body into high metabolic burn by eating protein rich food.

Q: Why is Emergen-C® fizzy drink allowed?

A: Most bariatric centers discourage patients from having bubbly carbonated beverages after surgery. The carbonation may cause discomfort in the pouch, may cause the pouch to expand temporarily and may cause temporary or lasting injury to the stoma. In addition, consumption of carbonated beverages generally means empty calories that are eaten with non-nutritional snack foods (think of the ubiquitous movie snack of a soda and popcorn). A fizzy vitamin drink mix is bubbly due to the effervescent reaction when the minerals react with the liquid. The fizz is not the result of pressurized carbon dioxide gas being forced into a liquid as is carbonation. Emergen-C® is an approved vitamin and mineral dietary supplement by most bariatric nutritionists. Some patients prefer to allow the effervescent bubbles to dissipate before drinking the vitamin mix. The rapid absorption of vitamins and minerals dissolved in water is an effective means for patients with malabsorption to take vitamin supplements.

Q: Does coffee count as water?
A: No. Coffee is coffee. Water is water. Coffee is a diuretic and will slow weight loss. Water will flush toxins and waste from your body and facilitate weight loss.

Q: How can I avoid constipation on the 5 Day Pouch Test?
A: Here are some ideas:

- Eat 1/2 apple with skin for your mid-morning and mid-afternoon snack
- Increase your fluid intake
- Include a water-soluble fiber supplement in your daily diet
- Add a fish oil capsule to your diet
- Drink herbal tea containing senna leaf in a small portion (6 fluid ounces): it is a powerful natural laxative.
- Prepare one of the Feed the Carb Monster Soups for days 1 & 2 (each 1-cup serving contains 5 grams dietary fiber). Look on the Internet 5daypouchtest.com or in the 5 Day Pouch Test Owner's Manual for recipes.

Q: Can I do the 5DPT Monday-Friday and then take weekends off?

A: No. That is not the 5 Day Pouch Test. The 5DPT should be used to break a processed carbohydrate addiction and get back on track with the high protein diet basics prescribed by your weight loss surgery center. You should follow the 5DPT and proceed with Day 6 following the basics of the DAY 6 DIET program outlined in this book. The 5DPT should only be used

in emergencies. See the topic "24/7? But Wait! I'm going to Maui!" in Part II
DAY 6 DIET Basics.

**Q: Do I need to follow the liquid restrictions when I have protein
shakes or soups on Days 1 & 2?**

A: Yes. Please observe the liquid restrictions for two reasons. First, even
though protein drinks and soups are liquids you do want to give your pouch
plenty of time to begin digestion and absorption of nutrients before
washing them through to the small intestine with liquids such as water.
Secondly, you are returning to the habit of liquid restrictions and this is a
good place to start. Keep an eye on the clock beginning on Day 1 and by Day
5 you will be in the grove.

**Q: Should I take my vitamin and mineral supplements while doing the
5 Day Pouch Test?**

A: Yes, please take your regular vitamins during the 5 Day Pouch Test. If you
have been taking them regularly continue to do so, between meals, with
water. If you have not been taking vitamins regularly wait until 15 minutes
after a meal and take them with a small amount of water so the remaining
food in your pouch will buffer them. Do not take them on an empty
stomach.

**Q: I am 13-years post-op. Is it too late for the 5 Day Pouch Test to work
for me?**

A: It is never too late. Give it a try. It is only 5 days. What have you got to
lose, besides a few pounds, that is?

**Q: Does my pouch really shrink back to the size when I first had
surgery?**

It is not so much that your pouch shrinks; it is that your pouch is not
stretched out as much as you felt it was. When we eat slider foods and
disregard the liquid restrictions, we do not enjoy the benefit of a tight
pouch. We feel it has stretched back to "normal" size because we can eat so

much more. By following the 5 Day Pouch Test and returning to a diet of lean protein, avoiding processed carbohydrates and slider foods and observing the liquid restrictions, we again enjoy the benefit of the small surgical pouch. It feels tight again the way it did after surgery because we are following the dietary guidelines that work with the tool, not against it.

Q: Is the purpose of the 5DPT to get in the mindset where we were when we first had the surgery?

A: That is absolutely a key purpose of the 5 Day Pouch Test. I don't care what it is in life, sustaining long-term enthusiasm for something can be strenuous. Look back at your life: have you seen hobbies or interests come and go? So here we sign-on to this weight loss surgery gig which at first feels much like a new hobby. We immerse ourselves in total learning like we would a new hobby. Then we find our comfort zone. Then we get bored and we find new interests, in part because of the freedom our new healthy WLS-hobby gives us. Our interest in WLS wanes. But unlike a fleeting hobby we are committed to WLS for the rest of our lives Employing the 5 Day Pouch Test to rekindle the fires of interest, excitement and enthusiasm is a great use of the resource. We invested so much of ourselves to have this new life; we must do whatever it takes to stay engaged in living well after weight loss surgery.

PART II: DAY 6 FUNDAMENTALS

*The vision must be followed by the venture. It is not enough to stare up the steps - we must step up the stairs. --
Vance Havner*

CHAPTER 4: DAY 6 DIET BASICS

We have found a new way to look at DIET, we have reviewed the Four Rules and we have reviewed the 5 Day Pouch Test. We find ourselves at Day 6. Day 6 is for the rest of our lives. The term "Day 6" self-evolved in the LivingAfterWLS Neighborhood after the surge in popularity of the 5 Day Pouch Test. So many Neighbors bonded in a collective effort to make the correct dietary, fitness, and lifestyle choices following the 5 Day Pouch Test that all days thereafter became Day 6. We often assure one another; Day 6 is the way we will live for the rest of our lives.

If you are looking for a chart or a list that details what food to eat at what time of day followed by the next food at the next time of day you will not find it here. Regimented diets served only one purpose in my life: they caused me to be morbidly obese. Strict diets, as I shared in Part I, do cause weight loss. But the minute I stepped out of bounds the lost weight came back and it brought friends. How many of us arrived at morbid obesity by way of the lose weight – gain weight highway?

I can recall, during my dieting career, discovering the latest greatest dieting miracle and reading with great faith programs that promised rapid weight loss by following a formula. For example, eat a grapefruit at 9 am followed by a piece of wheat toast at 10:15 and a glass of water 20 minutes later and another 3 pieces of grapefruit at 10:55 etc. and lose 2 pounds by morning. You get the idea. (Did you try something similar?) What a miracle! And I followed those silly programs to the letter! But the thing is, there is no miracle formula. If there were a miracle formula 60 percent of our population would not be overweight or morbidly obese and there would not be a half-million people a year undergoing metabolic and bariatric procedures.

Day 6: Beyond the 5 Day Pouch Test is not about magic tricks or secret formulas. It is not a regimented plan of strict do's and don'ts. Day 6 is a commonsense approach to making the most of your surgical weight loss tool so that you feel healthy: mentally and physically on most days. It is the act of treating yourself kindly by observing the DAY 6 DIET Creed: Daily Intelligent Eating Triumphs.

In this first section of DAY 6 DIET Basics we review simple things that make a big difference in our ongoing quest for wellness with surgical weight loss. Some of these hints may have been mentioned in passing during your early weight loss surgery education; some of them you may have learned in support groups or online. And maybe some of these hints are brand new. When you feel yourself veering from course give a quick review of these basics. I know I rethink the basics frequently and I'm often surprised how easy it is to forget that which works.

As you review the basics you have two opportunities to treat yourself kindly. First, when you read one of the Basics and think, "Yeah, right, I know that. I'm already doing that," do not dismiss this fact. Give yourself a big happy pat on the back and say, "YES! I am doing that! I am doing the right thing!" How often do we truly take a chance to congratulate ourselves on doing the right thing? If I were there with you I would be all over you with hugs and praise saying "Good for you! I am so proud of you!" Next, if you come across a Basic where you could improve here is your chance to try just a little harder and do just a little better to treat your body well. Make a mental note to pay more attention to the liquid restrictions or manage your fork just a little smarter. These are opportunities to excel, to treat yourself kindly, to improve your quality of living. Seize them!

Some Somber Thoughts. For the most part my intent with Day 6: Beyond the 5 Day Pouch Test is to uplift your spirit and inspire you. But I would be remiss if I failed to discuss the somber reason we had weight loss surgery in the first place and why it is essential we work diligently to keep our weight under control. Obesity has become a worldwide epidemic, encompassing approximately 1.7 billion individuals. Worldwide, more than 2.5 million obesity-attributed deaths occur each year. In the United States alone, there are estimated nearly 400,000 annual deaths due to obesity, second only to those due to smoking. Only 1 in 7 obese individuals will reach the US life expectancy of 76.9 years; the morbidly obese will live much shorter lives. Through aging, the quality of life for the morbidly obese is significantly diminished by grim co-morbid conditions.

Obesity is killing us pound by pound. According to the American Society for Metabolic and Bariatric Surgery about 15 million people in the United States have morbid obesity; yet only 1% of the clinically eligible population is being treated for morbid obesity through bariatric surgery. How is it that as a society we tolerate a system that allows 99% of the sick and dying to go untreated?

Surgical intervention has been shown to achieve long-term weight control for severely obese individuals. However, to ensure success, surgical intervention must begin with realistic goals and proceed with diligent behavior modification on behalf of the patient with long-term follow-up. According to a 2007 report published by SynerMed Communications®, "Bariatric surgery has been shown to be the only available effective therapy for severe obesity. Patients who undergo bariatric surgery typically experience substantial weight loss and resolution of obesity-related comorbidities. However, surgery alone is not sufficient to cause this weight loss. For successful and prolonged weight loss, the patient must fully commit to and participate in lifelong changes in his or her dietary habits and lifestyle. Without effective lifestyle management, the patient may not reach reported levels of weight loss regardless of bariatric technique. Effective management is a multifaceted process that includes medical, psychosocial, and nutritional factors."

Obese Elite. We are the fortunate elite of the obese, if there is such a thing, because we did have surgical intervention called "the only effective therapy for severe obesity." Sadly, this multifaceted lifelong approach described above is lacking and the stewardship of our surgical tool ultimately lies solely with us down the road after bariatric surgery.

I do not know where the blame lies, or if there is blame to be placed. But I do know that come three, five, and ten years or more out of surgery few of us have the multifaceted benefit of health management that includes medical, psychosocial, and nutritional care described above. In fact, nearly everyone I talk to describes the same scenario: "my primary care doctor doesn't understand weight loss surgery; I don't have a nutritionist; I am no longer in contact with my bariatric center; I am all alone."

The burden of stewardship is ours to bear alone. Perhaps the day will come when the ideal of multifaceted health management is realized. But until then we must diligently forge our own path. It is no wonder we are drawn to online communities for fellowship and advice. I know my greatest personal empowerment has come in learning from others who are part of this tribe. And we, like the penguins I spoke of in Part I, are a huddled mass counting upon one another for our very survival.

On this somber note let's move forward with our discussion of the things we have the power to do daily to ensure each Day 6 hums the sweet song of success.

SURGERY IS ONLY A TOOL

I smile when I say this because after 20 years it sounds like the greatest understatement in the history of the entire universe. But if you were naive like me you sweetly nodded your head in agreement when your surgeon told you prior surgery, "Now Kaye, this surgery, it is only a tool in your overall weight loss and weight management program." Who was he kidding? I was secretly hoping that it was my cure-all and I would never have to diet again. So, the joke was on me! He gave me my tool and then he sent me right back out there into the world that made me fat in the first place. Some joke.

> *"The patient should be made to understand that he or she must take charge of his own life. Don't take your body to the doctor as if he were a repair shop." --Quentin Regestein*

We take our new tool and all our curiosities and return to our same house and same job and same friends and same life. Nothing in our environment changes. The only thing that has changed is the quality and quantity of food we can eat and the way our body absorbs and uses that food.

Surgery does not take away a lifetime of learned eating behaviors nor does it automatically give us the knowledge, ability or desire to change the behaviors. It does not necessarily give us the confidence to defend our right to be nutritionally healthy to those who, even well intentioned, may derail our best efforts to follow the rules. It does not bring about a magical moment when exercise is fun. It does not condition those around us to respect and support our new lifestyle. It does not take away the lifestyle habits that corroborate unhealthy eating and sedentary living. We still go to movies, attend family celebrations, suffer from stress, keep over-booked calendars and we still get hungry. And guess what? We still love food. So it seems a cruel trick to get this "tool" and go right back to the world that made us fat.

To succeed with weight loss surgery, we have no choice but to make lifestyle changes. This is non-negotiable. Every lifestyle change that we affect in conjunction with "the tool" must be hard fought and purposeful. Lifestyle change does not happen easily. At times trying to do the right thing is painful and agonizing. At times it feels like the weight loss surgery we fought for has become a punishment. At times it feels lonely trying to affect positive health changes in a world where it's easy to be fat. And I'll be honest, there have been times I wanted to take my "tool" back and cash in on the warranty.

The only warranty; the only lifetime guarantee we get with this tool is the one we, the owner of the tool, are willing to endorse. When we sign the dotted line that gives another human being permission to trespass our body to manipulate vital functions and organs, we become the warranty holder of the results. No matter how difficult the challenges, how frustrating the change, we gave permission for this to happen. We are responsible for the tool now. We cannot change the environment into which we bring our new tool; but we can certainly heed responsibility and manage it to the best of our capabilities on any given day.

> *"If people knew how hard I worked to get my mastery, it wouldn't seem so wonderful at all." --Michelangelo*

Find your mastery. If you find yourself depreciating your surgical tool consider this: in 1508 Michelangelo di Lodovico Buonarroti Simoni was commissioned to paint the ceiling of the Sistine Chapel in Rome, Italy with a simple tool: the paintbrush. When placed in the hands of one who properly cares for the tool and works with steady attention to use it properly great things may be accomplished. Michelangelo was originally commissioned to paint the 12 Apostles on the ceiling; but at the completion of his work there are over 300 figures depicting numerous biblical scenes. Michelangelo used his simple tool, the paintbrush, and he exceeded his commission tenfold.

Do you have the enthusiasm to lovingly use your tool to get your mastery? As obese people we channeled great energy into going above and beyond in so many ways to prove we were more than our overweight bodies said we were. Channeling that energy to use our tool in a grand and abundant fashion is justice served.

I can eat anything I want. Remember in Part I where I shared the story of a person who laughed and said, "I can eat anything I want, just less of it?" Over the last ten years I've had a love-hate relationship with this sentiment. In the beginning I loved the idea that I would be able, after weight loss surgery, to eat anything I wanted, and the tool would do the work of keeping my weight under control. Later, when I learned this was false, I hated the statement and loathed the person who made it. I couldn't eat anything I wanted: I was working hard at weight control; the tool was not doing all the work for me.

These days, I accept the statement "I can eat anything I want." You see, I can and do eat anything I want. It is just that the things I want to eat have changed. They are not the same things that morbidly obese me wanted to and did eat. They are the things that healthy and aware me wants to eat. I chose to eat apple slices with a thin smear of peanut butter. I chose to enjoy lean grilled fish rather than battered and deep-fried fish. And give me green tea on ice with a twist of lemon over diet cola any day of the week, thank you very much.

Yes, I eat exactly what I want to eat. It is extraordinarily liberating to understand that we can eat anything we want after weight loss surgery and that we are empowered to make intelligent *(remember the "I" in DAY 6 DIET)* choices.

STOP BANGING YOUR HEAD!

My friend Jennifer is raising a daughter who is severely autistic. Her daughter suffers from intense headaches to which she responds by banging her head into the wall (Jennifer puts her in a helmet at the onset of these headaches). These episodes are so dramatic and distressing and Jennifer often finds herself saying to Rosie, "Rosie, if you continue to bang your head on the wall, you will continue to have a headache." Of course, reasoning is impossible at this point, but the example of Jennifer and Rosie illustrates what we, as recovering obese people, often do to ourselves.

> *If we continue to eat the things that led to our obesity in the first place, we will continue to be obese. If the behavior does not change, the result will not change. "Doing the same thing over and over again and expecting a different result is the definition of insanity." --Albert Einstein*

It is as simple as that. Today I can safely say that I can eat anything I want because my behavior has changed and the food I want to eat is different from the things I ate that caused me to be obese. It was a long way getting here. But it is a good place to be.

I imagine you are sitting there thinking this is all well and good that we change past behaviors, but how do we change the things we want to eat in a world where it is so easy to keep doing what we have always done? I expected you to ask that; you are an intelligent being seeking knowledge and that is why we are spending time together.

This is not new. Remember, you started changing your mind about the things you want to eat the first day you considered undergoing bariatric surgery. When that light went off in your head you said, "Enough! I no longer chose to live this way and I'm willing to take permanent and drastic action to change things." You looked yourself square in the mirror and made a promise for change, and you meant it. You loved yourself enough to sacrifice the things in which you once found comfort in order to become healthy, improve your longevity, and restore your self-esteem. There is not one single morsel of food on this planet that can give this to you.

Secondly, as a matter of practicality, the foods that once made us feel comforted are most likely to make us feel uncomfortable after surgery. If we had a malabsorptive procedure sugary carbohydrates and simple carbohydrates will cause dumping syndrome. High fat foods will also cause dumping syndrome. In a less immediate response sugar, starch and fatty foods will cause weight loss to cease or weight gain to occur. In addition, there is the mental torment that comes when we make poor food choices. Don't you wish you had a dollar for every time you made a less-than-stellar food choice and then beat yourself up for it? I would be a wealthy woman myself if I had a dollar for each poor food choice and the subsequent self-scolding! Recall in Part I the Dropped Egg allegory. When we make a poor food selection, we enter the cycle of one bad choice leading to another bad choice: we break all the eggs. By the end of the day we have really given ourselves a beating.

STAY ON PAR: PLANNING, APPRECIATION, RECEPTIVENESS

To lose weight and maintain a healthy weight we know we must change our diet from the things that made us obese and we must avoid eating things that cause us physical and mental discomfort. I offer my acronym PAR: Planning, Appreciation, Receptiveness; as a quick reference when you feel yourself straying from the path:

Planning: *verb* – to formulate a scheme or program for the accomplishment or attainment of a goal

For best results: plan meals and food selections. Whenever possible avoid leaving mealtime to chance. Plan generalities and "what if" scenarios so that you have rehearsed different life situations to avoid surprises. We have lived the routine of our lives for quite some time, we know at which events there will be food pushers and food police. Be prepared and have a plan.

One of the reasons the 5 Day Pouch Test is so successful is because for 5 days the plan is highly structured. We can do anything for five days, right? Of course, this is the reason some skeptics have called it a "crash diet." When we take the structured principals of the 5DPT test plan and adapt them to our Day 6 we keep the momentum of the plan, we retain the structure that keeps us on course, and we are spared the trauma of happenchance.

For me, a simple planner such as that shown below, works the best. As you can see, this menu is not overly specific, but serves as a rough outline taking into consideration different circumstances that are likely to occur in everyday living. Leftovers are introduced back into the menu rotation as lunches: cook once – eat twice! In addition to maximizing cooking time leftovers are saved from being lost in the refrigerator only to be found and wastefully discarded when they are past their prime.

On hectic days this plan makes use of ready-to-drink protein drinks or protein bars (Look for ready-to-eat protein products with 15g protein or more and fewer than 8g net carbohydrate). As we review this rough plan we know to make hard-cooked eggs for Monday and Thursday. We know to shop for salad greens, tomatoes, apples, grapes, melons and fresh produce. From our refrigerator, pantry, freezer or the supermarket we will need eggs, cottage cheese, chicken, ground meat, canned tuna, deli turkey, cream cheese, protein bars and drinks, and salmon. In creating a weekly menu we can reduce the number of trips to the supermarket, spend less time shopping and waste less money on unplanned purchases. We therefore have more time and money to enjoy living.

If planning three meals for seven days is too much to begin with start by planning just dinner meals. That is only seven meals a week. As your comfort level increases add lunch to your plan making use of the wonderful leftovers from dinner. Soon you will find breakfast falling into place.

A friend and fellow gastric bypass patient became quite frustrated with me as I explained planning meals to him. Larry griped, "What if I don't feel like eating grilled salmon on Friday? So much for your plan!"

I understand that a myriad of circumstances may warrant a change of plan and I respect that detours will happen. Honestly, I've arrived at Friday and not been in the mood for grilled salmon. But even in the face of change we are bound by the DAY 6 DIET creed to make intelligent dietary choices so at the end of the day we triumph. Change the plan if you must: just make your change intelligent. Swap out the salmon for sirloin and you triumph: swap out the salmon for beer and cheese fries and you have missed the opportunity to triumph.

Remember, every Day 6 requires a plan, and it can be your plan, your way. As I wrote on page 48 of the 5 Day Pouch Test Owner's Manual, "There are two things I know about human nature. First, nobody ever wakes up and declares, 'Today is the day I will relax my enthusiasm and get off track.' Second, nobody ever wakes up and gets back on track without first saying, 'Today is the day I get back on track and I have a plan.' Falling off track happens without a plan or script. Getting back on track requires a conscious decision, a carefully designed plan, and the determination to make it happen."

WEEK OF: _____   MEAL PLANNER

MONDAY	SHOPPING LIST:

MONDAY

TUESDAY

WEDNESDAY

THURSDAY

FRIDAY

SATURDAY

SUNDAY

SHOPPING LIST:

....
....
....
....
....
....
....
....
....
....
....
....
....
....
....
....
....
....
....
....
....
....
....

Meal Planner: You can download this worksheet, and all worksheets in this book for free at 5DayPouchTest.com. Click the Downloads link. LivingAfterWLS recently introduced a new line of life planners bespoke for the weight loss surgery patient. They address our special dietary and health management needs and focus on the long journey, not just a quick trip to goal weight. We want to stay on track for life and these planners are terrific tools to keep us on point. Find them exclusively on Amazon in print format. See my author page for a current catalog of all our publications.

Kaye Bailey Amazon page: https://www.amazon.com/-/e/B00LWITO8I

Appreciation: *noun* – to value greatly; gratitude, grateful recognition.

Perhaps I'm getting a little older or a little weary, but it seems of late as a society we are becoming increasingly cynical. Good manners have been usurped by trash talk and sarcasm. Respecting our elders and those in authority is the pre-historic behavior of fuddy-duddies.

By now you know me well enough to see that I'm a perpetual Pollyanna and I'm confident a whole lot of people these days find that annoying. So be it; I shall not be deterred. I believe in the good in people, I trust that most of us are doing the best we can on any given day to make the most of our life. I believe we are grateful for weight loss surgery and the opportunity to be healthy vibrant beings.

We are familiar with the expression, "If you seek fault surely you will find it." Years ago, during a dark time in my life I was quite capable of finding fault in many things and many people. The burden of cynicism was heavy and unbecoming: I did not bear it well. I don't recall the circumstances that led to a reversal in my thinking; but I do recall that when I sought things for which to be grateful surely, I did find them. My burden was lightened.

So here we are at the "A" in our PAR: Appreciation. It is so simple but oh so essential that we practice appreciation daily for all that is right and good in our lives. Did you know that psychologists have concluded it is impossible to feel gratuitous and begrudged at the same time?

When we empower ourselves with appreciation, we release potential we don't even realize we have. During any given week I get two different letters about the 5 Day Pouch Test. One will read: *"Dear Kaye, I am so grateful to have found the 5DPT; I am so thankful to think I can use my tool again."* The other will read: *"Dear Kaye, what if the 5 Day Pouch Test doesn't work for me?"* Who is off to a better start? Who has harnessed their inner potential?

Listen to the words your inner voice speaks to you and hush the voice that utters jaded negativity. Make a conscious choice to replace negativity with appreciation: the two cannot co-exist. Shout from the rooftops the words of the voice that proclaims gratitude. Deliberately practice the art of appreciation: it will keep you on PAR.

Receptiveness: *noun* – ready acceptance of new suggestions, ideas, influences, or opinions

I have a classmate from high school, Jerry, who through his own experience with a heart transplant now operates a home for people in the process of receiving lifesaving organ transplants. Terminally ill people, whose only hope of survival is an organ transplant, come from far and wide with their families and stay in his home awaiting the ultimate do-over at life. Another person's demise becomes the terminal person's second chance at living. Politics, religion, opinions, and habits: all checked at the door. It's a clean slate: the ultimate rebound.

In a way, perhaps to a less dramatic degree, weight loss surgery gives us a do-over at living. Surgery gives us a new infant-like stomach, a cleansed palate with new instructions, a new owner's manual, and a full serving of optimism. Every new post-op patient I met promises to "get it right" this time. We vow to follow the rules and pamper the new pouch and make right our gastric wellness as we conquer the disease of obesity with the best solution modern medicine can provide. And in earnest we try.

The surgical weight loss patients who fair best are those, who like the transplant patients, check all their pre-conceived notions at the door. Upon exit with our tiny new tummies, a cleansed palate and brand-new book of hope we take home an ideal of receptiveness that prior to surgery had long been dulled. The receptive post-op is willing to exercise despite unpleasant physical education memories. They are eager to try unfamiliar food or curious food combinations such as protein and fruit. They think outside of the breakfast box and eagerly enjoy a morning meal of tuna patties and tomato slices. Their receptiveness allows them to accept compliments graciously even if inside it feels awkward and unfamiliar. Receptiveness means embracing the awkward and unfamiliar because this is the ultimate do-over. And what is the point of a do-over if we are going to do the same thing we did before?

I cannot think of a finer example of receptiveness than the international soup sensation: Low-Carb Pumpkin-Sausage Soup from the 5 Day Pouch Test. This odd combination of ingredients that at first glance begs an incredulous *"what!"* has earned a cult following elevating it to "souper"-stardom and modest YouTube fame. And the Neighbors are eating it for breakfast! Just look what one Neighbor, Meg, said, "I just finished my morning bowl of the pumpkin sausage soup and it IS GOOD!! I hate diet food, have my whole life but this stuff is fabulous!" and Cheryl chimed in, "I made the pumpkin sausage soup tonight. Yummy! I'm going to have a hard time keeping the guys from eating my soup. This sounds so weird and tastes so good. It's very satisfying and filling."

This is exactly the kind of receptiveness I'm talking about: and it is not just about food. Consider exercise or new life experiences. Earlier this year my older brother, Jeff, known in the Neighborhood as Ambassador of Adventure, did the bungee jump off of the Victoria Falls Bridge on the Zambia - Zimbabwe border in Southern Africa. As a morbidly obese person suffering complications of sleep apnea and osteoarthritis this feat would have never been possible. Damon, our Neighborhood Godfather and extreme athlete, routinely races in century cycling events: 100-mile bicycle races in a matter of hours in all kinds of weather climbing and descending elevations that would make an obese man cry.

The ladies are equally receptive to adventure. Kim stomped grapes with her bare feet in wine country California. Darling Gwenda from Australia sneaks out at night to go Aussie Bush Dancing: I think there is fire involved. And Nancy in California is one hot lady riding high on her own Harley Hog.

Planning – Appreciation – Receptiveness: Let's stay on PAR!

Upcycle Your Head Hunger

One of the most popular buzzwords in the weight loss surgery vernacular is "head hunger." Commonly it is used to describe mental feelings of hunger for food versus physiological feelings of hunger. I dislike the use of "head hunger" in this manner and I think it sells short the momentum we can harness from a different kind of "head hunger."

Prior to surgery as we embark on the process of research into an effective treatment for our disease, we are the most voracious head hungry people you ever want to meet. We ask questions, we seek knowledge, and we dream dreams. Frightened be the man, woman or institution that gets in our way: we are head hungry for a release from the disease that is robbing us of our life. We are not lackadaisical in our approach to a surgical cure: we are full steam ahead. That is head hunger. It is also called determination.

And then, after surgery, mainstream media wants to turn us barracudas into whining babies crying, "I'm hungry for my pasta and my cookies and my ice cream." Message boards tell us in the days and weeks following surgery we should be "Head Hungry" for the same foods that made us fat in the first place. No thank you.

Head Hunger, to me, is that fighting grit determination within that says I will do everything in my power to make the most of this opportunity to be healthy and well. As we learned earlier, the recovering obese fortunate enough to be treated with surgery are the elite. It was because we were head hungry enough to fight for our right to be healthy that we had surgery in the first place. Head hungry for pasta or cookies? I don't think so. Head hungry for living? Absolutely.

A woman came to me one day, crying and suffering so called head hunger something fierce. I asked her, "Ellen, what has caused this reaction? Why are you so upset today?" She explained she had come to my office directly from the supermarket where she had wandered through the bakery looking at the pastries she could no longer have. Then she wandered the ice cream aisle looking longingly at the ice cream she is now "forbidden" to enjoy. "Why would you do that?" I asked? She explained, "Because I am four-months out of surgery and that's when we're supposed to get 'head hungry,'" she grieved.

Hogwash. As humans we are vulnerable to the power of suggestion. What if on that same day I had taken Ellen to a fashion boutique at the mall where she discovered a blouse two-sizes smaller than the one she was wearing fit her beautifully? Would she be wailing over ice cream and pastries? Or would she be doing the happy dance and celebrating her new life and wonderful shrinking body? You see the illustration here.

I will never indulge the popular "head hunger" theory in the manner it is perpetuated on many Internet support sites. I do not find it helpful or productive. The mind is a powerful thing and we can better use that power when we harness "head hunger" for the accomplishment of our healthy goals facilitated by weight loss surgery. And the best way to do that is with Double-D Action (DDA):

Distance & Distraction Action: Distance and Distraction Action must be employed when a trigger threatens to derail our best efforts of Day 6 living. Ellen would have been better served with DDA: going to the mall and trying on clothes to help her see that she was indeed accomplishing her weight loss goals. It would have done so much more for her mental health than perusing the bakery at the supermarket. And imagine the power of head hunger to continue following the Four Rules and the DAY 6 DIET Basics when she had physical proof (the size of a new blouse) that she was doing the right thing and her efforts were bringing about the desired results.

Ellen is not entirely to blame for her sorrowful wanderings in the land of forbidden food. We are subjected daily to retail manipulation that is the product of corporate investment and scientific study. The retail industry knows what pulls our triggers. Sights, smells, sounds, and product placement are not happenchance. They are the tricks of the trade that call us to action: the action of trading cash for goods or services.

And we cannot escape this retail manipulation: it is ubiquitous. Television and print advertisements beckon; aromas entice; and iconic brands elicit memories and trigger hunger. We go out the door to face the day and our only weapon against science and corporate spending: willpower. In the game of life willpower is not much good for armor.

You already have in your bag of tricks PAR: Planning, Appreciation, Receptiveness. That is a good start. Those are pro-active strategies. The DDA, Distance and Distraction Action is a retreat strategy. Move away from the war zone: you do not have the appropriate armor to survive and you must retreat. Retreat is to move back in the face of enemy attacks. Retreating means you know when to cut your losses and run for your life. There is no shame in receding to find safe harbor elsewhere: save yourself from harm.

Distance and Distraction Action (DDA) does not have to be as dramatic as all that, however. It can be as simple as putting down a magazine full of food happy advertising or taking a different path home to avoid and resist the pretzel vendor on the corner. We can defend against retail implosion by deliberately putting triggers out of sight and out of mind.

Sadly, sometimes our greatest battles are fought on our own turf at home and in our places of work. Those closest to us may unknowingly, or perhaps a bit on the sly, try undoing our efforts toward our healthy lifestyle. Just as we practice DDA – Distance & Distraction Action – with retail America, we must also practice DDA in home field battles. These are the most difficult of all. Advance reconnaissance could include making known our expectations before conflict arises such as setting boundaries. Request that your co-workers do not offer you sweet break room snacks, and then thank them when they respect you, don't pout or feel left out.

Advise family members that while you know they enjoy salty snacks you are no longer able to be the person responsible for stocking the pantry with such snacks. Respond to the family food pusher repeatedly with "No Thank You," as many times as necessary. Don't bother explaining yourself, food pushers do not listen, they are all about themselves.

Be consistent with your expectations, with your response when expectations are met and when your expectations are gone unheeded. The degree of your consistency will net a greater degree of respect in return.

A Perfect WLS Day

What if we had a sure-fire strategy to start the day with four easy actions that support our big picture goals of weight loss and weight management using the WLS tool? If we've already accomplished four simple actions in favor of a good day won't those help shield us from the bumps and bruises of the daily "broken eggs" (see Chapter 1: "Dropped Eggs Happen") we are bound to encounter? Check out these easy, quick, and affordable things we can all do to prepare the way for a perfect WLS day.

One: Breathe & Stretch. When was the last time you treated yourself to a good stretch upon waking? Are you like me, hit the alarm and hit the ground running to get to your busy day? Try this tomorrow morning as you wake to greet the day. Before rising take some big inhales and slow exhales: Oxygen is the energy of life. Studies suggest that deep breathing contributes to a longer life, and improved mood, stress reduction, and the release of harmful toxins. With deep breathing the blood becomes oxygenated which improves all functions in the body including the metabolism of nutrients and vitamins: So important after WLS. Further studies suggest that extra oxygen from deep breathing burns excess body fat more efficiently thus leading to improved weight loss. What a great benefit from a free and painless task!

Next stretch your limbs and body to loosen the muscles and open the cells to receive this healthy oxygen. Our cats already know that a good leisurely stretch is the best way to wake from sleep, we can learn by their example. A good morning stretch does not have to be the formal stretching that comes after exercise class. Think back to kindergarten when we stretched tall to touch the sky and bent low to touch our toes. Now sway left to right, right to left like a tree in the wind. Rotate your head and stretch your neck and spine. By now your good mood morning is underway and you've barely stepped out of bed! It's not just your imagination either: Stretching encourages the release of endorphins, providing a sense of tranquility and euphoria. You are now chemically predisposed to having a good day!

Two: Drink warm lemon water. Make no mistake, I love my morning coffee. But I know that my best days start with a warm cup of lemon water. Warm lemon water is an energy booster; provides hydrating electrolytes in the form of potassium, calcium and magnesium; reduces inflammation; improves digestion; helps regulate bowel movements; strengthens immune system; improves mood while reducing depression and anxiety associated with potassium deficiency; and improves weight loss by suppressing hunger cravings. Is it any wonder that cleanse programs prescribe warm lemon water first thing each day?

Warm Lemon Water is easy to prepare. Add 8 ounces warm (not boiling) water to a mug, add 1-2 tablespoons 100% pure lemon juice* and sweeten as desired with honey, agave syrup, or preferred beverage sweetener. Drink warm.

*I use ReaLemon 100% Juice from concentrate most of the time. While freshly squeezed lemon juice is delightful it takes an extra step in squeezing the juice vs. a quick pour from the bottle. At times fresh juicing is an inconvenient barrier. The juice concentrate removes the barrier and the excuse. Do what works for you!

Three: Eat protein. We know the first rule of weight loss surgery is to eat protein first. That means we must eat protein at every meal. The high protein or protein first diet is prescribed for all bariatric procedures and is the dietary guideline patients are instructed to follow for life. The bulk of our calories at any meal should come from animal, dairy, or vegetable protein. This includes breakfast. By eating protein first thing in the morning we instantly raise our metabolism, we promote feelings of satiation and reduce cravings for snacks or simple carbohydrates.

Eating a high protein breakfast effectively staves hunger cravings and snacking binges later in the day because it reduces the circulating levels of the hormone ghrelin, which stimulates hunger. So not only are we raising our metabolism with high protein nutrition, we are managing the brain chemistry that often gets the blame for head hunger and snacking binges. The earlier in the day we eat protein the more likely we are to stick with our high protein diet plan without annoying cravings or sluggishness.

Try starting your day with 35 grams of high-quality protein including eggs, meat, poultry, shellfish or fish, Greek yogurt, milk, cottage cheese, vegetarian protein, or protein supplementation such as protein shakes or protein bars. I keep hard-cooked eggs on hand for a quick-grab breakfast and habitually mix my ready-to-drink protein shake with hot coffee (use it like coffee creamer) for a steady supply of morning protein. For more protein breakfast ideas check out Breakfast Basics:

Four: Plan a treat. In a perfect world we all make a weekly menu, do the shopping and preparation, and stick to our plan like NASA scientists. Then there are the rest of us! Sometimes my best effort is to plan the next meal and even getting that done is a chore. But on my best days, if nothing else, I plan a meal that I can look forward to when thoughts of food sneak uninvited into my day.

So much of our food psychology is looking forward to a meal or treat in association with an occasion. By providing a meal or treat to look forward to we acknowledge that core human desire to anticipate sustenance. We provide opportunity to feed the psyche and soul as well as the biological necessity for nutrition. With the help of weight loss surgery, we are mindful of our choices ensuring they support our health goals. It is a matter or re-allocating those basic human behaviors in a manner that supports our greater goals. And by starting each day with a plan for one meal --*one moment of reward and enjoyment*-- we can easily harness those behaviors to benefit our health rather than contribute to our illness (obesity).

Here ae a few treats I look forward to eating:

o Fruit and/or berries with dairy protein (yogurt, cheese, cottage cheese)

o Ready-to-eat shrimp and cocktail sauce

o Pickles with Cheddar cheese

o Avocado with chopped hard-cooked egg and diced tomato. Add salad greens or seasonal vegetables for a full meal.

o Turkey Roll-ups (Layer two turkey slices, smear with cream cheese and jelly, roll-up and refrigerate for a wonderful handy snack! Delicious beyond compare!)

o Cooking with Kaye favorite recipe: Light Fresh Turkey Salad

o Protein Pudding (Whisk together 1 package sugar-free instant pudding with 1 can ready-to-drink protein drink. Chill and enjoy. Use serving size recommendations on pudding mix).

o Warm herbal tea or chilled iced tea infused with lemon, berries, fruit, herbs or other seasonal flavor boosters.

LIQUID RESTRICTIONS

Gastric bypass, lap-banded, and sleeve patients are all advised to avoid drinking liquids 30 minutes before meals and 30 minutes after meals and no liquid with meals. The time restriction varies from surgeon to surgeon, but most use the 30 minutes before, 30 minutes after restriction. Follow your surgeon's specific directions. When the liquid restrictions are followed the pouch fills more quickly with less food volume. It stays full longer advancing digestion and the feeling of satiation is reported to last longer.

That makes perfectly good sense: so why are the liquid restrictions so difficult to follow?

Because, eating food without the lubrication of liquid makes us physically uncomfortable. We experience dry mouth and the pouch feels tight and compact. Conversation is difficult. And the pleasure of eating is short lived: four, five bites and we are done while those around us continue to have a jolly good time.

I believe that during a social meal the liquid restrictions may be slightly relaxed so we can enjoy ourselves and feel part of the conversation. Another post-operative patient taught me this little trick: between bites of food take a small sip of water and hold it on your tongue. Slowly push your tongue to the roof of your mouth pushing the water to the sides of your mouth along your checks then swallow. She convinced me that this small amount of moisture is just enough to coat the mouth for conversational purposes without completely violating the liquid restrictions. Try it now. What do you think? Do this only after every second or third bite or just before you wish to speak. It does make a world of difference.

Having practiced this technique for several years I report no adverse consequences and have happily enjoyed many conversational meals. It should be noted that I observe faithfully the liquid restrictions for private silent meals.

The other time when I feel it personally acceptable for me to relax the liquid restrictions is when enjoying a glass of wine or cocktail. Alcohol affects us quite differently after gastric surgery; this is discussed in the next chapter in detail. It is my preference to enjoy a short pour of red wine with a meal so that it is not as quickly absorbed, as it would be if taken on an empty pouch. Seek the counsel of your physician so you may make an informed personal choice regarding your alcohol consumption after weight loss surgery.

Ignoring the liquid restrictions causes the greatest problem when we bring slider foods (described below) into our diet. When liquid restrictions are abandoned, and fluids are used to wash down slider foods the effectiveness of the pouch is diminished. This is not a mealtime behavior lapse; this is a snacking or grazing habit combined with disregard for the liquid restrictions. Disregard of liquid restrictions combined with slider food consumption will most assuredly lead to weight gain, carbohydrate dependency, and psychological distress.

SLIDER FOODS

Conversationally have you ever let someone off the hook for doing something inappropriate by saying, "Don't worry: we'll let it slide this time," realizing of course you were actually meaning, "What you did was wrong but I will ignore it this time."

How interesting is this? We know when we eat processed simple carbohydrates (chips, crackers, cookies, bread, etc.) and wash them down with liquids that we are not following the Four Rules we agreed to upon accepting the lifetime terms of weight loss surgery. But we go ahead and "let it slide" this time. We ignore the fact that we are blatantly disregarding the rules. By ignoring the rules and eating slider foods we, figuratively and literally, let it slide.

Please imprint this in your brain to call upon in times of hesitation before reaching for slider foods:

Slider Foods = Letting it Slide

When you are compelled to reach for a bag of cheese snacks (my personal bad-carb beacon) chant in your head "slider foods letting it slide; slider foods letting it slide; slider foods letting it slide" several times over. I know, it sounds hokey, that's why I'm asking you to do it in your head, not out loud. The repetition of this simple message will override the environmentally triggered desire to eat non-nutritious food that falls in the snacking-grazing-slider food category. You already know when you are reaching for that bag of empty carbohydrates that it is not an intelligent dietary choice (DAY 6 DIET). This is just a mental string around your finger to reinforce why you deserve to make a better choice. Please don't dismiss this as silly, try it at least once, for me, please? The mind is a powerful thing: you are where you are today in large part due to a strong will of survival and grit determination. You have greater power than any bag of empty calorie snacks.

As a point of clarification, I am often asked if yogurt, soup, protein-fortified pudding, and whole grain breakfast cereal with milk are slider foods. This question is about the near-liquid consistency of such foods, which literally makes them slide. Two things will keep these foods in the meal category: nutritional content and measured portions. Slider foods are non-nutritious processed carbohydrate food eaten without regard to portion size or nutritional value and washed down the pouch and through the stoma (pouch outlet) with non-nutritious liquid in unmeasured portions. They are consumed mindlessly without awareness to volume or the specific deliberate intent to provide nutrition to the body.

It is true that yogurt, soup, protein-fortified pudding, and whole grain breakfast cereal with milk will pass through the pouch more quickly than solid lean protein and we will not experience the feeling of fullness as long. However, because these liquids contain nutrients, our bodies will continue to absorb vitamins and minerals from the food as it passes through the jejunum into the small intestine.

KAYE'S 2B/1B RHYTHM

I admit measuring food portions is a real pain in the kitchen! And it is near impossible in a restaurant. At home I know exactly which little custard cup holds a half-cup of cottage cheese and I use that same little bowl every time I have cottage cheese or yogurt. I know that a hard-cooked egg is 6 grams of protein. And I know that a serving of chicken breast is 3 ounces and should be about the size of a deck of cards. Wait! I don't play cards: how big is a deck of cards?

Measuring food and counting food grams feels tedious and confusing. Over the years I started playing my own game at mealtime and eventually it became the 2B/1B Rhythm that I have shared so often with the LivingAfterWLS community it has become a recognizable acronym by many. It simply means that when I'm eating for every two bites of protein, I take I follow them with one bite of complex carbohydrate. Hopefully a low-glycemic fruit or vegetable such as steamed green beans, grilled squash or peppers, or crispy salad greens. Because we do not eat fat in bites, I consider it incidental to the meal and do not concern myself with counting or fussing over fat grams or bites. This, of course, assumes that I have followed the DAY 6 DIET creed and intelligently selected a meal that has been healthfully prepared with an appropriate proportion of good fat.

I am not sure the nutritionists or scientists would be 100 percent in favor of this rhythm method. But then again, I know that I am more likely to practice this method of measurement than tipping the scale for each meal. I believe even this imprecise method is better than no method at all. I also find that if I follow the 2B/1B Rhythm I am more likely to experience fullness sooner than if I randomly pick at the food on my plate. As we know Protein First is at the top of our WLS rule list for a reason.

STARCH IS A CONDIMENT

It is no secret that Americans love our pasta topped with rich sauce and succulent meat. In fact, we love it so much major restaurant chains lure us through their doors with the promise of all we can eat pasta. I recall, back in the good old days before surgery, that on spaghetti night we brought out the big dinner plates and served abundant portions of pasta topped with a copious amount of sauce and cheese. And my goodness, we cleaned our plates soaking the last of the sauce with crusty garlicky buttered toasted bread.

Pasta was the food I expected to miss most following weight loss surgery. In fact, my final meal, my last supper if you will, was taken at a nationally known pasta house and I ate myself into carbohydrate slumber one final time.

Oddly, I don't yearn for pasta. In fact, it rarely crosses my mind and almost never winds its way around my fork. I've tasted a nibble here and there since surgery, but the texture does not appeal to me and it feels like a lump in my pouch that lingers long past its welcome. *(This is still true as I mark my 20-year milestone.)* I know other surgical weight loss patients who quite enjoy pasta and find it agrees with their system just fine. It is odd how we all respond differently, but then again, people with normal digestive systems have dissimilar responses to the same foods, so why should we be any different?

Regardless of our digestive response to pasta, or any other soft cooked starch such as rice, polenta, or grains we need to be cognizant of portion size. Overeating pasta will likely cause weight loss to stall and weight gain to occur because it is a simple starch easily converted to fat stored by the body. Next to slider foods, also simple carbohydrate, pasta consumption is a leading cause of weight regain in weight loss surgery patients. As you may be aware, when eating pasta there is a strong urge to have liquid with the meal for a more comfortable feeling, hence the liquid restrictions ignored. Ultimately, we consume a greater volume of non-nutritious starch.

A surprisingly easy action can prevent this pitfall. Rather than get out the big plate onto which we heap the starch serving first I suggest treating starch, especially pasta, as a condiment. Here's how: onto a small salad plate measure a 1/2 to 3/4 cup serving of meat sauce. Top with a 1/4 cup serving of pasta or starch and sprinkle with 1 tablespoon of cheese. This will reduce the simple carbohydrate intake significantly while providing the culinary enjoyment from a controlled serving of pasta or starch. It is the bite of the pasta we most enjoy, not the heavy feeling of overeating pasta. After the meal you will feel lighter and not suffer the carbohydrate slumber from pasta overdose.

BECOME AN ARROGANT GOURMET

For most of my life I thought fine dining meant eating at the food court, at the county fair and at the open refrigerator door. For me, good home cooking was hamburger skillet meals from a box "helper" mix or a casserole made with condensed soup and noodles. Sour cream solved any culinary crisis that Velveeta cheese couldn't correct. Eating directly from the container standing at the fridge was a beloved pastime. I ate with a shoveling deliberate intense motion because I was thinking about the next bite I'd stuff in my face, not the food presently in my mouth. I was an ugly eater and a poor home cook. And I was obese because of it.

After gastric bypass surgery not one of those behaviors could be indulged. Not one. Talk about a wake-up call! During the phase of rapid weight loss I ate a bland repetitive diet. I followed every rule, I achieved goal weight and I declared myself a WLS success. And then I went back to the kitchen to learn to cook. I was ready to eat again, but I was not ready to return to obesity. I wanted to cook healthy balanced nutritious meals so that I did not have to be afraid of food.

I started with one cookbook: The Cooking Light Cookbook, and read it cover to cover comprehending the healthy cooking tips and noting what appeared to be protein dense, flavorful, nutritious recipes. I learned cooking techniques. I experimented with different flavors and textures and with new ingredients. And during this period of learning I did not gain weight. Imagine, being in the kitchen, preparing food, sampling and dining and not gaining weight.

Some recipes were disappointments, most likely a failure of the cook. Some things made me sick; dumping and vomiting. I learned along the way and I kept trying new things. Recognizing a good "safe" recipe became easier.

But most of all, I became an "Arrogant Gourmet." I'm not talking about a hoity-toity foie gras' and truffles kind of nose-in-the-air gourmet. I'm talking about being discriminating with ingredients and selective with the foods I feed my body. I am no longer willing or able to eat copious amounts of nutritionally void foods of marginal flavor or quality.

TODAY I CHOSE NOT TO EAT BAD FOOD.

Weight loss surgery was my second chance at life, but it did not mean I would never eat again. It forced me to cultivate an appreciative palate favoring quality over quantity. It taught me to feed my body well. I never expected such a fabulous outcome from such a desperate solution.

One Bite Under Policy. As I became acquainted with my new gastric bypass pouch and advanced to solid protein I thought the objective was to eat until the pouch was full to capacity. More times than not this sent me to the bathroom because I had gone one bite too far and needed to relieve the pressure by vomiting. Time and experience have taught me to stop short of full: I call this the One Bite Under Policy. A full pouch is not comfortable to me, particularly if I have been stellar about following the Four Rules. Mostly protein fits tight in the pouch and it lingers, just as it is supposed to do. My slogan is:

One Bite Under – Just Right! Not too Tight!

To learn what one bite under feels like we must practice mindful eating at a slow and deliberate pace. Follow the 2B/1B rhythm and practice fork control (described below) between bites. Monitor the volume of food as it leaves your plate keeping in mind a visual of how much is in your tiny pouch. When you think to yourself "I know I shouldn't have this last bite" you have gone too far. If you think, "I could hold one more bite," then set your fork aside and wait a moment. I believe you will find you have arrived at a content and comfortable place. In twenty years of living after weight loss surgery I can honestly say I have never regretted the last bite not taken. It is the one bite over that begets remorse and penitence.

Fork Control. We have heard this nugget of dieting advice: put down the fork between bites of food. This is a tough habit to acquire and once acquired an easy habit to slip away from. Because of my work in the weight loss surgery field I consider the world my laboratory and, apologies extended, I often find myself studying strangers in public eating situations. Not long ago I observed a couple eating across the table from one another: she quite heavy, and as luck would have it, he quite thin.

During the the meal he spoke with great animation barely taking time to eat or breathe. She nary uttered a word, nor did she release her fork; it was an extension of her arm. As she worked each bite in her mouth she busily and intently loaded the fork with the next bite. I did not see her make eye contact with her dining companion. Not once. Perhaps she focused on her fork and food to suffocate his incessant droning about a topic in which she had no interest. Or perhaps she was absolutely captivated by the food upon her plate. I don't know the answer. But what I do know is that I remember being the woman with the perpetually loading fork as I mindlessly fed myself into oblivion.

It is basic. Put down the fork between bites. Concentrate on the bite in mouth and enjoy.

There is more to this DAY 6 DIET basic than simple fork control. Physiologically, when we put our fork down and do a complete job of chewing our food before swallowing, we advance the digestive process. This means we are giving our surgical gastric pouch a better chance to digest the food we are eating. Fork Control plays a key role in the One Bite Under Policy described above. And since we have made intelligent food choices it stands to reason we would elect to give our body the best opportunity possible to make the most of our intelligent choice.

WLS is 24/7? But Wait! I'm going to Maui! My sister Julie, who in her own right has been successful with a popular mainstream weight control program after bearing two children, taught me a powerful lesson about my own weight loss surgery. She and her family were preparing to vacation in Maui, Hawaii. She told me she would not be "dieting" that week; she had given herself permission to enjoy any food that struck her fancy. I was so excited for her: she had worked hard and she looked fabulous. Julie is fabulous! She then indicated, "It isn't like you. You have your 'diet' with you 24/7. You never get to take the week off and go to Maui and eat whatever you want." She said it so kindly and tenderly, it was not hurtful. It was matter of fact. She spoke the truth.

A popular mainstream weight loss program advertises, "Take weekends off!" The inferred message: if we are good (follow the program rules) during the week, then on weekends we are rewarded with a state of dietary anarchy where there are no rules. By Monday, after two days lived in the absence of any common dietary sensibility, we must start anew and repeat the cycle.

This is so popular that the diet "Cheat Day" is a celebrated thing, promoted by commerce and celebrated by misguided dieters. I find it absurd.

Can you think of another way to treat your body more unkindly? Okay, chain smoking, heavy drinking, and reckless driving: I get it. There are worse things we could do. But the nutritional chaos caused by this cycle is no doubt a leading contributor to the expanding waistline in this country and the growing mental despair we suffer as our health declines and we forfeit the motivation to keep trying.

Consider this example: Your daughter faithfully follows your instructions to wear her bicycle safety helmet on Monday, Tuesday, Wednesday, Thursday and Friday. Proud of her compliance, on Friday night you praise her, "What a good girl you have been wearing your safety helmet all week. This weekend, as a reward, you may ride your bike wherever you wish, and you do not need to wear your safety helmet."

No parent would risk their child's life to give them a "reward" so foolish. Why would we risk our nutritional wellness with the reward of dietary anarchy? Isn't the benefit of good health substantial reward in itself?

Our weight loss surgery is our 24/7 safety helmet. And aren't you glad? Look where "weekends off" got is in the national sport of dieting? Weekends off took us right to the front of the line of morbid obesity. Weekends off put us in the danger zone where we risked our lives. I want my weight loss surgery with me 24/7 because I like feeling safe.

NAVIGATING IN THE REAL WORLD: THE HOLIDAYS

One of the challenges we face with weight loss surgery is returning to the same environment in which we lived before surgery; the exact environment that contributed to our obesity. It seems to me there are more real world complications than I have coping skills. Let's look at some of those environmental complications and evolve some strategies to manage them without giving up the greater cause of health and recovery. For me the winter holidays bring the greatest challenges or should I say opportunities to work on my coping skills?

Feasting Season: During the feasting season –*Halloween through New Year's Day*-- it is very typical for magazines and news programs to report the calorie count of traditional holiday meals. The Thanksgiving Day Turkey Feast easily comes in at 1,400 calories and the Christmas Day Prime Rib Extravaganza packs in a whopping 1,800 calories. Experts warn us that weight gain from holiday eating is inevitable. But I dare say, it is not the big meals that do us in: it is the BLT's: Bites, Licks, and Tastes. I wish I knew which diet program or person coined the BLT's so I could give them credit, it has been in my diet-talk for as long as I can remember. You have probably heard it too.

The BLTs: The Bites, Licks, and Tastes will do us more harm than any big meal because even with our little tummy pouches there is always room for another Bite, Lick or Taste. When we sit down to a meal our pouch fills quickly, fullness is signaled by discomfort, and we stop eating. That is how the pouch is supposed to work. But standing in the kitchen stirring a sauce or baking cookies we always have room for little Bites, Licks and Tastes. I've talked to many people who are in the BLT boat with me, maybe you are there too. Here are a few tricks I've learned to help me avoid caloric uptick and weight gain that comes from unchecked BLTs.

Eating vs. Tasting: A skinny professional chef taught me this trick to use when preparing sauces, reductions and gravies. Good cooks know it is necessary to taste mixture for seasoning and texture throughout preparation. As a home cook my inclination is to use a soup spoon to take full spoonful of the sauce: That's a taste. "You are using the wrong end of the spoon!" the chef scolded. The skinny chef demonstrated that by using the handle end of the spoon and simply dipping the tip in the gravy for a taste on the tongue he could quickly discern seasoning and texture. This method provides the needed information at the cost of very few calories. "The objective is to taste mindfully and deliberately in order to make an informed decision about the sauce. "You, on the other hand," he said, "were eating, not tasting." What an awakening moment! He was correct. In fact, I am certain that in many cases I have eaten a meal's worth of calories in tastes.

Picky Taster: Some things simply do not require a taste test like pasta, rice, potatoes or other starchy side-dishes. Face it: we already know how pasta or rice tastes so when we taste-test pasta or rice we are either tasting to check doneness or we are eating. I realized most of the time my tasting habit is better described as eating. Skinny chef said he learned to test pasta and rice for doneness by taking two samples: one he would chew and the other he would cut with a fork on a cutting board. The simultaneous action of chewing and cutting taught him the feel of doneness with utensils so he no longer needs to taste for doneness. Now he only tests doneness with the fork and cutting board method. As he told me, "I'm in the kitchen for 10 or 12 hours a day. If I tasted a sample from every pot of pasta this kitchen puts out it would add up to hundreds of disappointing calories a day. I already know how pasta tastes. Why take on those calories?"

Spit like a lady: One of the most elegant sophisticated women I know has a job that requires her to taste-test food for a commercial retailer. On a given day she may be required to taste 12 cheesecakes and a dozen different cupcakes. Some job for a person recovering from morbid obesity with weight loss surgery! This classy woman has no qualms about tasting and spitting. She tastes, chews, and spits. This singular sample informs her opinion without derailing her steady dietary efforts. There is no shame in spitting. In that corporate tasting room these days she is not the only person doing the taste-chew-spit evaluation. Few of us have jobs with taste testing for a task, but we do have occasions when it would serve us well to spit. Just spit like a lady and carry-on!

Break the sweet-salty cycle: For me the sweet-salty cycle rears it's ugly head during the winter holidays. A handful of nuts, a bite of sugar cookie, pretzel sticks, gumdrops and on it goes. Are you experienced in the sweet-salty cycle? I recall that after meals my dad would say he needed something sweet to chase the taste away. After gastric surgery this eating cycle can be disruptive: it leaves me feeling wonky.

Recently I have adopted the French tradition of imbibing a palate cleanser between menu courses to remove lingering flavors in the mouth and improve digestion as well as prepare the taste buds to receive the next offering. A palate cleanser effectively stops a sweet-salty cycle. Granted, I don't enjoy multi-course meals often. What I have found is the palate cleanse works after eating to refresh and signal that the meal has come to an end. It is a simple and effective fix. Try iced water with a pinch of lemon zest and a squeeze of lemon juice stirred in with a little honey for sweetness. Or try green tea or mint tea, warm or iced, to break an eating cycle. It really works.

Practice Awareness: is perhaps the greatest weapon we have in the ongoing face of temptation by way of Bites, Licks and Tastes: Awareness that BLTs do contain calories and lead to weight gain; Awareness that weight management for those of us battling morbid obesity is literally a matter of life-and-death; Awareness that we deserve nutritional wellness that can only be achieved by the choices we make with our fork.

TIPS TO STAY ON TRACK IN THE FEASTING SEASON

Breakfast: Eat a protein breakfast first thing. A protein dense meal kick starts the metabolism: it also provides a feeling of fullness.

Water & Beverages: Drink 24 ounces of water between breakfast and your next meal or snack. A well-hydrated body works efficiently and reduces hunger cravings. Continue to drink water throughout the day: at least 64 ounces.

Appetizer Buffet: Practice the 2 Bite-1 Bite Rhythm (2B/1B) and liquid restrictions while partaking from the appetizer buffet. Specifically, eat two bites of protein for every bite of fruit or vegetable carbohydrate. If you are eating from the buffet avoid liquids until you have finished your food. Remind yourself by having a food plate or a beverage in hand, not both.

Slider Foods: Remember that crackers, pretzels, cookies and white breads are non-nutritional slider foods. If you give yourself permission to enjoy some of your favorites remember the liquid restrictions. Following the liquid restrictions will decrease the amount of processed snack foods we eat in a single sitting because there is nothing to wash them down. Even slider foods will help you feel full when observing the liquid restrictions.

The Big Feast: Get greedy with the protein; be stingy with the side dishes. I'm a sucker for the ubiquitous green bean casserole so I'll indulge with a bite or two on a special holiday. Treat yourself to a favorite dish and then let it go. It is just food. Remember your liquid restrictions but celebrate too. It is acceptable to take small sips of your beverage at a big meal. A moist mouth facilitates conversation.

Gatherings: Holiday meals and family dinners last a few hours; they do not last for weeks. When the meal is over, it is over. Remove your plate and avoid post-meal nibbles during kitchen duty. Better yet, let someone else do clean-up. Go for a long walk: assign kitchen duty to the kid table. Go ahead and say, "My doctor prescribed that I must walk after every meal, I'd love to help but it is important that I take care of my health." Leave the clean-up and the post-meal nibbling to someone else.

Dessert: Contrary to popular belief, food does not have morals. Desserts are neither good nor bad: they are just desserts. If you have a perennial favorite take a bite or two and savor the moment. Then let it go. Discarding something you chose not to eat is perfectly appropriate and sadly necessary. Discarding food at gatherings is risky business. I'm sure you can think of instances in your life where food rejection is tantamount to the eighth deadly sin.

Clever discretion is called for. Consider the options: spit in a napkin, stuff it in your handbag, feed it to the dog, "accidentally" spill your plate. All risky. None of us wants to hurt Aunt Edna's feelings: she is infamously proud of her holiday fruitcake. Besides, kindness and appreciation should never be on a diet. My favorite opt-out is to accept the offering and make it a "to go" treat for later. I then offer praise to Aunt Edna: I know how splendid her legendary fruitcake is, and I'm anticipating savoring it later when I'm not so full and thank you ever so much. Aunt Edna feels treasured and I have not betrayed my personal goals. Now that's a happy holiday.

The day after the feast: As should be our habit, start the day with a protein dense breakfast. Drink lots of water. Avoid slider foods. Take vitamins and medications as usual. Engage in the activities of daily living. Pat yourself on the back! You have the power to celebrate a feasting day without allowing it to become the launching pad for a six-week downward spiral of unchecked eating that leads to weight gain and poor health.

MY TIPS & TRICKS FOR THE FEASTING SEASON:

ARE YOU A FLATTERY-FLOOZY OR A YEAH-BUT-BETTY?

After attending several WLS events recently I started noticing a trend among our weight loss surgery sisters that may seem at first superficial but once examined reveals much about the emotional journey from obesity to healthy weight. Unlike other diseases, obesity can be observed and diagnosed by the lay person: men, women, and children alike. Who among us doesn't cringe at the memory of an innocent child drawing attention to the "Fat Lady"? While this lay-diagnosis is most often uncomfortable and probably unwanted, wearing our disease in our plus-size britches also provides opportunity for positive feedback when we are losing weight and becoming healthier. Feedback can be complimentary, "You look wonderful" or incredible, "You have lost a TON of weight" or nosey, "Did you get THE surgery?" or underhanded "Too bad you lost all that weight only to lose your hair and find all those wrinkles!" It's no wonder we evolve coping personalities to emotionally manage this feedback. As obese people we had coping strategies as well. Think of the forever funny fat lady who is really crying on the inside while laughing on the outside. She makes herself the target of her own fat jokes just to beat others to the punch and avoid the hurt.

I ask you to please forgive the gender bias in this article: I am addressing the female persuasion. Guys are different about man-to-man compliments. As my own big brother Jeff who is also weight loss surgery patient told me, "It goes like this: "Dude! You've lost weight." "Yeah." "Cool!" And there it ends. No baggage there, right?

With the ladies I find that two typical personalities emerge, see if you recognize them.

Flattery-Floozy cannot get enough of the compliments. In fact, she valiantly deserves an Academy Award for her weight loss "After" performance. Flattery-Floozy loves to receive compliments. It matters not the sincerity or authenticity of the compliments tossed her way. After years of watching life from Wallflower Alley she is blooming, and she is not going to miss a moment of it. Who can blame her? I recall feeling starved for compliments and attention after suffering the invisibility that comes with being overweight. I wanted to hear anything different from the feedback I'd heard all my life, "You have such a pretty face, if only you could lose the weight..." Flattery-Floozy loves sharing her weight loss surgery success story and loves the attention. She nurtures a sense of entitlement: it is her due after suffering from years of living in the shadows hidden by her own body.

Flattery-Floozy is likely to suffer a loss of pre-surgery friends who may feel betrayed by her weight loss, or they may accuse her of changing. She simply may no longer fit with the group. This does not make her a bad person, though her friends and peers may judge her harshly. It is simply the evolution of living, of change, and of growth. As detailed in an earlier chapter almost every WLS pre-op patient I speak with says, "I won't let the surgery (and weight loss) change me." But find that person a year or two down the road and they have changed significantly. So have their relationships. We are sometimes critical of this change. But I defend it saying perhaps this is the person we always were and now we have the confidence to bloom and thrive without the burden of disease. We no longer feel the need to hide.

Disease changes people and so does treatment and recovery. We are not critical of people who change as they travel the journey of other diseases. We empathize and accept them: they are seriously sick and working very hard to recover. Perhaps we can extend that same empathy and kindness to ourselves and others suffering and recovering from obesity. Even Flattery-

Floozy deserves some empathy and acceptance, especially as a gift to herself.

Yeah-But-Betty. Next we have Yeah-But-Betty. She is the opposite of Flattery-Floozy. Perhaps the years of feeling unworthy of attention or love or compliments have taken a toll. She feels undeserving and almost embarrassed to be noticed, as if she were granted weight loss by magic without investing her own blood, sweat, and tears. In response to a compliment you will almost always hear Yeah-But-Betty reply, "Yeah, but look at how much weight I'm still carrying on my belly" or "Yeah, but I don't think I can keep it off," or "Yeah, but I had the surgery to lose the weight." You will often find Yeah-But-Betty in an imaginary race with other weight loss surgery patients on the same timeline. Like the stat-riddled sports commentator she is ready with numbers, "Yeah, but at 6 months out Better-than-Me-Bonnie was down 100 pounds and here I've only lost 60 pounds." Yeah-But-Betty is never first to cross the finish line in this race.

We sense that Yeah-But-Betty feels she will never be good enough or deserving enough or accomplish enough to merit compliments and attention from others. She is loathe to treat herself to a few inwardly uttered positive words of self-praise. While Flattery-Floozy is likely to reinvent herself with a whole new look including wardrobe and hair style, Yeah-But-Betty continues to hide in shapeless clothing too big for her ever-shrinking body. In fact, I've met a few Yeah-But-Betty's still wearing their over-sized sweatshirts even after losing the weight of a super model. Nobody will take her to task for letting the weight loss change her. And she will probably keep her pre-surgery circle of friends. Hopefully they are supportive and complimentary of her new-found health by way of bariatric surgery.

I have not observed that one or the other personality is happier than the other. But what I know from my own experience and my work with so many of you is that both Flattery-Floozy and Yeah-But-Betty are terribly insecure. And this insecurity is not resolved with a flashy new outfit or by hiding in that comfy old familiar Winne the Pooh XXL sweatshirt. I don't necessarily believe that either personality needs to be corrected because this is part of the journey. But what I have learned is that the insecurity and self-doubt should be nurtured with self-kindness and compassion. One way to do this is invite Appreciation-Annie along for the journey.

Appreciation-Annie reminds us to stop for a moment, look where we are, and be in the moment: take in the experience. She understands that the journey: the experience is what life is all about. She knows in the big picture goal weight and all those surface milestones are really much ado about nothing. She is your best friend who never speaks ill of others and always has a kind word to share.

Appreciation-Annie is gracious in accepting compliments. Unlike Flattery-Floozy who flaunts her entitlement or Yeah-But-Betty who minimizes her accomplishments, Appreciation Annie considers a compliment a gift. You can hear her say, "Thank you for saying such a nice thing to me, it means so much to me to hear it coming from you." Like Annie, you would never dismiss a gift offered you by saying, "Yes, I deserve this!" or "Yeah, but, I am not deserving." We know that is bad form and insulting to the presenter of the gift. Accepting compliments is as much about respecting and appreciating the giver as it is about being a deserving and gracious receiver.

This single thing, the mindful act of appreciation, is a powerful builder in mending the frays of insecurity. In appreciating compliments and good health and little moments we begin to realize we are deserving. Make every season one of good will, giving, and receiving. And the greatest kindness we can accomplish begins from within.

UNDERSTANDING HUNGER: LEARNING THE SIGNALS

Hunger is not the only physiological signal managing our food intake. There are several factors that decide when it is time to eat and when it is time to stop eating. As recovering morbidly obese people it is important to understand the signals our body sends in order to lose weight and not become morbidly obese again. After all, ignoring these signals contributed to our obesity in the first place. (The following definitions are from Understanding Nutrition (Whitney & Rolfes, 2005), pages 252-256).

Hunger: the painful sensation caused by a lack of food that initiates food-seeking behavior.

Hypothalamus (high-po-THAL-ah-mus): a brain center that controls activities such as maintenance of water balance, regulation of body temperature, and control of appetite.

Appetite: the integrated response to the sight, smell, thought, or taste of food that initiates or delays eating.

Satiation (say-she-AY-shun): the feeling of satisfaction and fullness that occurs during a meal and halts eating. Satiation determines how much food is consumed during a meal.

Satiety (sah-TIE-eh-tee): the feeling of satisfaction that occurs after a meal and inhibits eating until the next meal. Satiety determines how much time passes between meals.

There are three types of influences that trigger hunger: physical, sensory and cognitive.

The most reliable influence is physical: an empty stomach, gastric contractions, and the absence of nutrients in the small intestine, gastrointestinal hormones and endorphins. Sensory influences such as the thought, sight, smell and taste of food will trigger hunger. And finally, perhaps the influence we know best, cognitive. That is the presence of others, special occasions, perception of hunger (head hunger), the time of day or the presence of food. In other words, external cues.

But as we all know, there are mental and external cues that can lead to hunger, appetite, and even satiety. According to Understanding Nutrition,

"Eating can be triggered by signals other than hunger, even when the body does not need food. Some people experience food cravings when they are bored or anxious. In fact, they may eat in response to any kind of stress, negative or positive. These cognitive influences can easily lead to weight gain." (Whitney & Rolfes, 2005)

As we go forward with our post-surgical weight loss living it is important to pay attention to the feelings of satiation and satiety. The small stomach works well (when used correctly) to signal a feeling of satiation and indicate it is time to stop eating. This leads to satiety, which is like a pink sticky note that reminds us to not start eating again.

Develop a new awareness and listen to your body. Finally, just as hunger is not an emergency, it is also not a failure. If you feel hunger during the 5 Day Pouch Test carefully assess the signals to decide the state of urgency. After careful assessment if you are still hungry then eat something from the approved list of foods for the day. Associating hunger with feelings of failure often leads to destructive eating and inappropriate food choices. Feeling hunger is not a moral problem: it is simply a small part of a very complicated biological process.

HUNGER IS NOT AN EMERGENCY

It was about a year after my weight loss surgery that my mother sent me my baby book. What a treasure to receive. In that record of my early life I read that as an infant I cried frequently at length but could always be soothed with ice cream. How interesting that as an infant my comfort was found in high-fat sweet carbohydrate deliciousness. Reading that gave me pause to consider how often over the years I have reached for food without exploring what else my body may be craving. I think many of us have been conditioned to reach for food when our body is sending distress signals without discovering what exactly it is that the body is distressed about.

114

Needful Pings: I no longer call the signals "hunger pangs" I call them "needful pings" because my body needs something and it is pinging me, much like the Blackberry does when it calls for attention. The Blackberry has different sounds for different needs: How nice it would be if the body was so clever! Alas, it is ours to learn with each needful ping what our body needs. There are four non-caloric responses that I find effective in soothing the body: I call them Four First Before Food: oxygen, hydration, wiggle therapy and rest. Below I describe each response and why it works.

Oxygen: Slow, deep abdominal breathing can lower blood pressure, slow heart rate, and relax muscles. The functional purpose of breathing is to draw oxygen from the air into our lungs. The oxygen passes to the red blood cells, which oxygenate all cells of the body. Upon exhaling we release carbon dioxide waste.

In Bharti Vyas' book: Beauty Wisdom: The Secret of Looking and Feeling Fabulous" she writes, "Good Breathing, and for that matter good, clean air, floods our cells and tissues with dynamic oxygen which has the power to galvanize cell metabolism and boost cell turnover. The benefits are immediately noticeable in the freshness of our skin tone and the brightness of our eyes. And because everything is ticking over efficiently, we feel more alert and alive."

Experts agree taking a 5 to 10-minute breathing break can be more refreshing than taking a nap. Find a calm space to sit or lie down. Close your eyes and focus as you inhale and exhale naturally. Do not exaggerate your breathing, just focus on slow steady deep breathing. The quieter: the better. Continue to observe your breathing until this deeper slower rhythm becomes automatic. Stop when you feel your strength returning.

Healthy breathing is as much a part of our healthy living after weight loss surgery as diet and fitness. By focusing on our breathing, we can improve the flow of oxygen and prevent internal pollution, both of which have a dramatic impact on the way we look and feel. Just breathe.

Hydration: Here we are back to the raw basics: Rule #2 – Lots of Water (See Part I – the Four Rules). The body does not readily discern the difference between a cry for food and a cry for water. We have discussed the benefits of water. To make things more interesting let's consider adding a squeeze of citrus to our water, or perhaps some frozen berries for a chilled drink. Herbal teas are soothing. They have natural cleansing properties and antioxidants that keep our immune systems healthy. Diluted fruit or vegetable juices are also a fine source of hydration.

Avoid liquids that are carbonated (we will discuss this in the next chapter), contain caffeine and alcohol. Rather than satiate thirst they act as diuretics and often trigger hunger pangs.

If you are a new post-operative patient, particularly a bypassed patient, be mindful of water and liquid temperature. Colder water causes the stomach muscles to constrict and tighten: this is uncomfortable. Banded patients will notice a tightening of the band when cold liquids are consumed. Find your comfort zone and stick with it: this will help you enjoy staying hydrated.

Wiggle Therapy: They taught us wiggle therapy in kindergarten and it worked wonders on our tiny little bodies and developing brains. And then we got all grown up and sophisticated and forgot all about it. It is time to bring it back and I love it! Let me refresh your memory, but first put yourself back in kindergarten: maybe you are sitting on the rug and story time has just concluded. Your teacher, the one you just adore, says, "It's time to shake the wiggles out!" And at once 25 little kids jump up from the rug in crazy wiggly-jiggly-giggly good time fun. Remember that? Why in the world did we give that up? We put our arms above our heads and reached for the sky. We bent down and touched our toes. We hopped, skipped, wiggled and jumped. There was not a self-conscious wallflower among us. We were silly wiggle worms.

I suppose wiggle therapy takes about a minute, maybe less. But the effects are lingering. Better than a chocolate buzz, the wiggle thrill lasts for quite a while. Our thoughts become clear and our focus sharper because we have joyously told our metabolic workers inside, "There is a party going on outside!" Our heart rate is elevated, and our blood oxygen levels increase. And the needful ping we may have perceived to be hunger is gone.

Now, realistically, in a grown-up society I know in many cases it would be frowned upon to leap up from our work-a-day to gyrate about in wiggle therapy. No doubt we would be committed to another kind of therapy. However, in a more subtle fashion we can stretch, flex and bend our bodies delivering respectable doses of oxygen to the cells while causing a meaningful rise in heart rate. And if all else fails, make haste to the rest room and lock the door. Then go crazy and shake the wiggles out.

By the way, if you are an office worker tethered to your desk all day there is a legitimate health reason to practice wiggle therapy. Extended time seated in an office chair increases the risk of deep vein thrombosis, a condition that causes swelling, pain, and potentially fatal blood vessel damage. Inactivity slows circulation, which can lead to a blood clot. Protect yourself with a session or two of wiggle therapy each day.

Rest: In Part I we talked about our collective trait to be nurturers and care givers. Routinely we will sacrifice sleep so that we may better spend our time caring for others. As our body becomes weary we tend to mistake its cry for respite as a cry for food. Thinking back to my infancy as recorded in my baby book I wonder how many times I cried and was fed ice cream when what I really needed was a nap.

As an adult one needful ping I once thought was hunger is often a cry for rest. I put rest as the last of my "Four First" because it is the most difficult to accomplish in an adult world. Oh, to be back in kindergarten. Story time, wiggle therapy and now, how about a nap? Good times.

Resting does not necessarily mean slumber. Rest, the verb, is to take repose by ceasing work or other effort for an interval of time: relax, unbend, and unwind. During the workday that may mean stepping away from technology and turning away from our tasks for a defined amount of time. Health experts agree that a 10 to 20-minute break from the demands of the moment is effective in restoring energy and mental focus.

In an ideal corporate world management would give a nod to science and call time out for napping each afternoon. A cyclical dip in body temperature has been found to occur consistently between 1 and 3 PM prompting researchers to recommend a 10-20-minute nap around 2 PM. In studies such a nap has proven to boost alertness for several hours and increase productivity.

The environment in which we chose to take our repose is critical to the success of the act. We must extricate ourselves from all disruption. Perhaps you have a nearby outdoor space where there is peace. A dark vacant office can serve as a place of technology-free intermission while you ponder and collect your thoughts. And in desperate moment, having worked many years in the corporate world, I concede to taking my fair share of respite breaks locked in a bathroom stall simply hoping for 10 undisturbed minutes to myself.

Care should be given to our evening rest habits as well because they directly affect our health and wellbeing, and even our weight control. We may think of sleep as a luxury, but it is a mandatory way to improve our health and it should rank as high on our priority list as taking our vitamin supplements, following the four rules and annual check-ups.

As we listen to, respond, and respect our needful pings our bodies will become stronger and we will be more in tune with them. This harmony will serve us well through life.

ACCOUNTABILITY: BE YOUR OWN HEALTH GUARDIAN

Since its introduction in 2016 the LivingAfterWLS Personal Self-Assessment Worksheet, shown on the previous two pages, has proven to be effective in prompting the enthusiasm and behaviors that support our long-term weight loss goals. As I mark my 20th' anniversary of gastric bypass I continue to schedule and complete this form once a quarter. (Hint: Schedule time for the worksheet on your digital calendar and set it to repeat every 90 days. Keep this appointment the same as any health management appointment.) I treasure that the worksheet can be a pat on the back when I'm doing well and the kick in the derriere when I'm struggling. I share this tool with in in hopes you respect the task as you evaluate goals and identify opportunities for improvement. Start today. A year from now you will be glad you did.

Your completed worksheets should be saved for reference. Dedicate a binder for your paper worksheets or file them digitally as you build your personal archive of accountability. What we have learned is the people who do a regular self-examination (every 3 months) are less likely to wake-up a year down the road only to wonder how in the world they have gone so far off track.

It is important to keep in mind the Self-Assessment is not about perfection and this is not a graded task. You are your own health guardian and this tool provides opportunity and space to honor a contract with yourself to stay on track and continually work at living a healthy well-guided life. I've been doing this assignment for many years now and what I know is that it isn't always easy for me to complete this worksheet each quarter. Like you, I can be relentlessly hard on myself. But what this exercise teaches me, time and time again, is that despite my insecurities most of the time I'm making progress and I'm willing to keep leaning and keep trying. Health management and weight management is hard. We may naively think the work is done when we get to goal weight or somewhere thereabouts. But there is no finish line in this race, not until we take our last breath and our body goes cold. That is how harsh the reality of weight management is.

This living after WLS is challenging. If you are in maintenance now you understand how truly difficult weight and health management is. You probably also realize that you are left to your own devices to manage a complicated disease. That's why you are here. Connecting with others who understand is a terrific resource in a world where we may feel let down by the medical establishment. Do you know that most WLS patients lose contact with their bariatric centers as early as three years after surgery? Our general care doctors don't really understand us and conventional weight loss programs snub us for taking the "easy way out" by having surgery.

Perhaps you are asking "What's up with all these worksheets? Why do you nag me about keeping records so much?" I get it, and sometimes I think if I'm given one more form or survey or worksheet, I'm likely to stab my eye with a factory sharpened No.2 pencil! I get it. But you see, time marches on and what happened last week or last month fades. If we notice a weight gain, we can return to our personal health file and look at what we were doing differently when we were losing weight. How many of us benefit from that EUREKA! moment when we realized we've started drinking liquids with meals and can eat oh-so-much more than when we were not?

Hope and desire are false-heroes in the tale of life-long healthy weight management. I dare say if hope and desire were all it took for us to lose weight and keep it off bariatric medicine and the weight loss industry would be naught. Remember the planning phase before your surgery: Did you have hope and desire to spare? And soon after surgery reality manifests:

hard work and steadfast effort fueled by the hope and desire was the new normal. Think about it: having weight loss surgery only to come back to the world that contributes to our obesity is the Mt. Everest of health management. We aren't going to get to the top of that mountain on hope and desire alone – if that were true would you have submitted to major

120

surgery forever rearranging your digestive system? Nope, we would have boarded that plane called "Hope & Desire" and soared to the mountain top.

The self-assessment allows you to harness the energy and enthusiasm of hope and desire to fuel the hard work and effort required. Additionally, your completed worksheet validates your worth. You deserve to take time and evaluate your health. You deserve to set goals, articulate them, own them, and achieve them.

Finally, if I can use one more metaphor, the worksheets allow us to see the forest through the trees. Countless people have thanked me for the Self-Assessment because this tool is tangible evidence of progress. We often learn we are doing better than we thought. In general, overweight people are harsh in their personal assessment. We see flaws and failure so easily. But when we take the time to put on paper the honest answers to critical questions, we often learn we simply aren't doing that badly. Do the self-assessment and see yourself in a new light. It is empowering to look back and see on paper just how far we have come. I know you are doing better than you think you are doing. Let's find out!

Quarterly Personal Self-Assessment

Date:

The LivingAfterWLS "Quarterly Personal Self-Assessment" tool is a worksheet of questions we can ask ourselves in a sincere effort to assess our present state and make an action plan for the next three months. This worksheet should be used as a private tool with the intent to keep your eye on the goal. It is a contract with yourself; a contract of honor and self-respect because you deserve to treat yourself well and engage in appropriate long-term behaviors in pursuit of your healthiest life. Please accept this invitation to join me in the Quarterly Personal Self-Assessment. Take some quiet time to evaluate where you are and where you are going. Commit your WLS goals to paper. Pre-ops, Newbies and Old-timers all benefit from the use of this tool. You can do this. *Always review your previous quarterly worksheets as you begin this exercise.*

Body: I am physically: and this is supporting/disrupting my healthy efforts.

        I weigh: and I'm [ ] LOSING [ ] GAINING [ ] MAINTAINING.

Mind: I am mentally FOCUSED/DISTRACTED regarding my WLS experience.

        My thoughts are:

Heart: I am socially and emotionally HAPPY/SAD which is positively/negatively affecting my well-being.

        My relationships are:

Write a personal assessment briefly summarizing your overall health and wellness pertaining specifically to your obesity management with weight loss surgery:

My top 3 goals when I had WLS were:
        Indicate if they are ONGOING (O) CHANGED (C) or ACHIEVED (A)
        1)
        2)
        3)

In pursuit of these goals list the strengths and strategies that are contributing to favorable results:

As with any journey there are struggles. Where have you struggled and what improvements could be made to produce better results?

Copy & Use this worksheet. Download all Day 6 worksheets as printable files at 5DayPouchTest.com

Define the goal you will pursue this quarter. Why is it important and worthy of your energy and effort? Does it contribute to your long-term health and weight management?

Including your strengths, knowledge, abilities, and intentions define your approach to achieving this goal. Map a strategy for each barrier.

Make a commitment.
Based on the assessment above I will:

The specific tools/methods I will use for my success are:

Will I enlist the help of others? Who/What:

Make your agreement binding:
My next appointment for self-assessment is: _____ (see page 135)

In solemn contract with myself I hereby agree to honor these commitments:

_____
Signature & Date

CHAPTER 5: KNOWLEDGE BASE

This is the textbook section of our Day 6 living. I have chosen these topics because they address the concerns we share. Perhaps you have wondered about alcohol, caffeine, carbonation, nutrition, sugar, and revisions. Those topics and others are covered here. Many include links to Internet sources so you may continue to study things that concern you after weight loss surgery. What I present here are topics I consider most important: the things I regret not having more information about which may have prevented all those extra lessons at the school of hard knocks.

IT'S NOT ABOUT VANITY ANYMORE: OBESITY IS A DISEASE

Many factors influence body weight—genes, though the effect is small, and heredity is not destiny; prenatal and early life influences; poor diets; too much television watching; too little physical activity and sleep; and our food and physical activity environment. --Harvard School of Public Health

In June 2013, the American Medical Association (AMA) made headlines when its governing body adopted a policy that recognized obesity as a disease requiring a range of medical interventions to advance obesity treatment and prevention. Previously obesity was considered a condition resulting from behavioral and environmental factors and a contributor to other diseases rather than a stand-alone disease. This new designation produced passionate opinions both in favor and against categorizing obesity as a disease, and the debate continues a year later. People in favor of the disease designation say it brings attention to the intervention, prevention, and treatment of a debilitating metabolic disorder. Opponents say calling obesity a disease overlooks the dominant effect of lifestyle choices that contribute to obesity, specifically food intake and energy output. Both schools agree that obesity is a complicated health problem with factors of genetics, biology, environment, social, and behavior all playing a role.

What I know about the weight loss surgery population is that understanding and accepting obesity as a disease is crucial in our individual approach to lasting weight management with surgery.

WHY I ACCEPT THAT OBESITY IS A DISEASE

First: Medical intervention for a medical condition. I must accept that obesity is a disease because in 1999 I consented to go under general anesthesia so a surgeon could cut-and-paste my digestive system in a fairly new radical abdominal surgery (Lap-RNY). I conceded to this desperate intervention and treatment of my chronic obesity in order to improve my health and longevity that was otherwise catastrophically compromised. It is impossible to reconcile having major life-changing abdominal surgery for the purpose of correcting lifestyle choices or habits, or to make a cosmetic improvement to body weight for the sake of vanity, don't you think?

Second: Medical conditions merit serious attention and care. If I have a medical condition that is being treated with surgery and lifestyle changes then I must take seriously the post-surgical protocol and make my health management a priority. Obesity as a disease takes our perception beyond the glossy headlines "Eat less, move more, lose weight." Obesity as a disease opens the door for understanding that a comprehensive approach to treatment must be ongoing and include resources such as nutritionists, fitness coaches, support networks, and medical and psychological wellness care.

Third: A medical condition is not a moral character flaw. Once we recognize the disease, we can separate from the self-defeating perception that we are the disease. We can change our language from "I am fat" to "I have obesity" which means something quite different. Obesity is a disease, not a definition. Once I remove the moral label and social stigma that comes with the words "I am fat" I can sensibly approach my treatment plan without the emotions of blame and failure that so often get in the way.

Fourth: Relapse and remission are part of the disease cycle. A disease is seldom cured but rather a disease is put in remission. A remission is a temporary end to the medical signs and symptoms of an incurable disease while a relapse is a recurrence of the past condition. A disease is said to be incurable if there is always a chance of the patient relapsing, no matter how long the patient has been in remission. For the person with obesity relapse is manifest in weight gain. Understanding this relapse as part of the disease cycle liberates us from moral blame and self-declared failure. We can marshal our resources and intelligently work toward remission by making the lifestyle changes necessary with the support of our medical team.

I AM ME; I AM NOT MY DISEASE

o   Obesity is a disease.

o   Weight loss puts the disease in remission.

o   Weight gain puts the disease in relapse.

o   As with most diseases, those who suffer obesity are responsible to make dietary and lifestyle changes that work in tandem with medical treatment to keep our disease in remission.

o   Like most diseases, relapse occurs and obesity manifests relapse with weight gain.

- We are never limited in the number of times we can actively affect behaviors to put obesity in remission: we always have another chance.
- Most importantly, I am not the disease, I have the disease.

Many factors influence body weight—genes, though the effect is small, and heredity is not destiny; prenatal and early life influences; poor diets; too much television watching; too little physical activity and sleep; and our food and physical activity environment. -- Harvard School of Public Health

Assignment: How do you define obesity and what role does your thinking play in your overall approach to your ongoing weight management with surgery? Title a blank sheet of paper "My Thoughts on Obesity" and detail your view of obesity as you consider the personal, public, and medical aspects of the condition.

BEVERAGES: WHAT WE NEED TO KNOW

What's in your glass? Beverage rules and beverage consumption continue to be a point of confusion for many post weight loss surgery patients and with good reason. The information routinely provided at the point of surgery tends to be vague and inconsistent. Further adding to confusion are urban legends and tall tales shrouding all things liquid in a veil of mystery.

Here is what I have learned from research and experience about the effects of alcohol, caffeine, and carbonation on our bodies post gastric surgeries. These are generalities, of course. For your specific concerns please speak with your surgeon, bariatric nurse counselor or bariatric nutritionist.

Alcohol: Working in the weight loss surgery support field I read extensively the material bariatric programs provide their patients. The Frequently Asked Questions most always briefly address how alcohol will affect a person after a gastric bypass, banding or sleeve procedure. And without deviation the answer most commonly reads:

"You will find that even small amounts of alcohol may affect you more quickly than prior to surgery and higher blood alcohol levels will occur with smaller amounts consumed. Alcohol may be more toxic on your liver."

This generic answer hardly warrants notice. It is no surprise that many of us have found ourselves doing the walk of shame wondering why a few social drinks, that before surgery would have made us charming and delightful, now push us beyond the abyss of drunk and falling. Recently popular media has put the shame-blame on us saying we have transferred food gluttony for liquor lust. They call it "transfer addiction". I do not buckle to that blame because I have done my research and I understand the physiological response our surgically manipulated systems have to alcohol. I believe the following is what we should be told during our pre-surgical education:

Alcohol is a molecule, just two and a half times the weight of water. This little molecule requires little or no preliminary enzyme activity for digestion. Absorption into the bloodstream begins at first taste, in the mouth, and continues as alcohol travels down the esophagus directly into the stomach pouch. In that short journey of mere seconds 10 percent of the alcohol has been absorbed into the bloodstream. I often report immediate onset of wine glow with the first taste from my glass.

The alcohol continues to absorb through the stomach or pouch lining into the bloodstream, but at a slower rate. On an empty pouch, alcohol will flow through the stoma much like a low-flow faucet left running. The stoma from the pouch on a gastric bypass patient empties directly to the middle portion of the small intestine. Without the benefit of gastric enzymes, which are absent in malabsorptive procedures, alcohol is rapidly absorbed into the bloodstream at a rate as high as 75 percent.

Blood Alcohol Level (BAL), also known as Blood Alcohol Concentration (BAC), will rise at a dramatically rapid rate. In addition to the volume of alcohol consumed, the rapid rise in BAL is affected by other factors including body weight, body fat, age, gender, nutritional status, physical health, and emotional state.

Considering body weight, think back to how a frosty mug of beer or a glass of wine affected you prior to weight loss. Did you feel a buzz or a glow from one standard drink? If you have lost 50 percent of your body weight you have also lost 50 percent of your blood volume. That means your body has 50 percent less liquid with which to dilute the alcohol it has just rapidly absorbed. Simple math reveals the fact: one drink has twice the potency it did prior to weight loss.

Further complicating our ability to safely ingest alcohol is the loss of digestive enzymes that occurs with malabsorptive procedures, as mentioned earlier. Gastric surgery causes decreased activity of the alcohol-metabolizing stomach enzyme, alcohol dehydrogenase (ADH). Without ADH more alcohol reaches the bloodstream faster and intoxication occurs quickly. As vaguely referenced in the standard bariatric answer quoted above, alcohol consumption without the benefit of digestive enzymes may lead to alcohol-induced liver and heart damage.

Sounds serious, doesn't it? Reviewing the physiology of our re-plumbed digestive system clarifies our understanding enabling us to avoid alcohol overconsumption. Knowledge gives us the power to make intelligent choices about our alcohol intake and avoid moments of shame and embarrassment that we may otherwise not understand.

Research suggests we are well advised to drink controlled portions (3 to 5 ounces) of alcohol only after a meal that includes fat, protein, and carbohydrates. The alcohol will mix with the food molecules and slow the rate of absorption as the chyme (partially digested semi-liquid food mass) passes through the stoma and enters the middle section of the small intestine through the stoma. We are advised to avoid alcohol consumption in quantity and never drink on an empty stomach pouch. This rule holds true for all bariatric and metabolic procedures.

Ongoing studies are beginning to indicate that surgical weight loss patients who do not practice controlled alcohol consumption may build a tolerance for it and later develop a dependency upon alcohol. Please exercise caution in the consumption of alcohol after weight loss surgery and always seek the advice of a qualified health care provider.

Carbonation and Caffeine: Like our pre-operative question about alcohol, we are told to avoid beverages containing caffeine and carbonation without the sensibility of further explanation. Here is what my research has taught me and why we should avoid both carbonation and caffeine in our post-WLS diet:

Carbonation- Carbon dioxide is added to a liquid to produce bubbles making an effervescent beverage such as soda pop or soft drinks, sparkling wine, beer and seltzer water. After the carbon dioxide is added the beverage is

packaged and sealed, and the carbon dioxide remains inert until opened and atmospheric pressure acts upon it causing bubbles to be released. The bubbles are called carbonation.

In drinking carbonated beverages atmospheric pressure continues to force bubbles to be released from the liquid even as it makes its way from our mouth through the esophagus and into the stomach pouch. This release of carbon dioxide will put pressure on the pouch causing it to expand temporarily. If we are eating while drinking carbonation our pouch will hold more volume than normal because of the enlargement that results from the temporary stretching. More damaging, however, is that the release of carbon dioxide bubbles may force the food through the stoma and over time the stoma will enlarge. Eventually the stoma will not recover from repeated enlargements due to protracted consumption of carbonation. Weight gain will occur because food will flow too quickly through the pouch and satiation will not be achieved.

Caffeine – Beverages that contain caffeine include carbonated soda, coffee, tea and some sports stimulant drinks. The primary reason to eliminate or reduce caffeine from the diet after surgical weight loss is because it reduces the absorption of calcium into the body. Studies have found that caffeine increases urinary calcium content, meaning that high caffeine may interfere with the uptake of dietary calcium into the body.

Caffeine found in coffee and tea tends to cause an increase in gastric acids, which may cause discomfort for some bariatric patients. In addition, caffeine is a diuretic causing water loss due to frequent urination, which may lead to dehydration. Additionally, patients who tend to drink beverages other than water tend to fall short on their water intake.

NUTRIENTS, PROTEIN, CARBOHYDRATES, FAT

I am not particularly comfortable giving specific one-on-one nutritional advice to my weight loss surgery Neighbors. First, I'm not a health care worker so I'm not qualified to render such advice. Secondly, I cannot see you to make a semi-informed analysis of your health. Nutritional advice is serious business and should only be given after verbal consultation and laboratory blood analysis, always with trusted health care providers.

What I can do here is provide you the current generalized recommendations, so you have a point of reference when speaking with your qualified health care provider. We may not always have the luxury of speaking with our bariatric centers, so it is wise to educate ourselves on the current bariatric standards and practices of nutrition.

In general, based on the broad-canvas study, bariatric centers agree patients should follow a 1,200-calorie a day diet. The protein, fat, and carbohydrate recommendations are based on that recommendation.

Protein: Common recommendation for daily protein intake is 60 to 105g (20-35% of a 1,200-calorie diet). Protein digestibility and quality are important factors that patients must consider when making food or supplement choices. The digestibility of protein is increased when accompanied by a full array of vitamins and minerals.

Fat: Fat is necessary for the growth and development of the basic components for hormones, skin, hair, transportation of fat-soluble vitamins, and insulation and cushion for the body and internal organs. As a rule, the bariatric profession abides the American Heart Association recommendation of 27 to 47grams daily fat consumption in a 1,200-calorie diet. It is beneficial to take fat-soluble vitamins with food sources that are rich in mono and polyunsaturated fats such as avocado, tuna, salmon, olive oil, flaxseed, and canola oil.

Carbohydrate: Carbohydrate provides the body with its preferred source of fuel and is the only source of energy for the brain, central nervous system, red blood cells, kidney, and retina. Bariatric patients are counseled to choose complex carbohydrates over simple carbohydrates. Bariatric centers do not generally recommend a specific daily carbohydrate allowance, according to Swilley. The report referenced the generally accepted recommended intake for all people provided by the National Academies' Institute of Medicine of 113g carbohydrate consumption daily in a 1,200-calorie diet. It is unlikely a gastric surgical patient of any procedure could meet this recommendation.

VITAMIN AND MINERAL SUPPLEMENTS

The report also looked at vitamin and mineral supplementation for patients. Her findings identified no clear results as she states here, "Surgery creates an increased risk for deficiency of certain nutrients. Decreased intake in combination with varying degrees of malabsorption presents unique challenges to achieving the macronutrient and micronutrient status needed to thrive. Lifelong preventative actions, such as supplementation, regular follow-up, and thorough patient education are mandatory for accomplishing all the benefits and avoidance of the health risks involved in bariatric surgery. Given the nature of the procedure and the individuals undergoing the procedure, no clear protocols have been determined. The focus, therefore, is on risk reduction and careful monitoring and follow-up, versus risk elimination."

Supplementation: As Swilley states in the report summary, no clear protocols have been determined due to the nature of the surgical procedures and the variety of individuals undergoing the procedures. The topic of supplementation, based on theory, opinion, and postulation becomes quite divisive among weight loss surgery professionals. There are differences and confusion for those of us on the front lines as well when we compare notes with what we have been told, what we have read, and our own experience.

However, there are three supplements universally agreed essential to our nutritional balance: daily multivitamin; B12 supplement; and calcium citrate. Iron and magnesium are frequently prescribed for bariatric patients and briefly detailed here.

Daily Multivitamin: Bariatric patients are advised to take a daily multivitamin in liquid, chewable or powder form that contains the Recommended Daily Allowance (RDA) levels of iron and zinc. The UL for iron is 45mg per day for adults and the RDA for zinc is 12mg for women and 15mg for men.

B12: The commonly recommended dose of B12 is 500 to 1,000mccg per week delivered via an effective absorption route (i.e., sublingual tablet, nasal gel, or B12 patch) or 1,000mcg IM once monthly. Blood lab work is the only effective method of measuring B12 values in the body.

Calcium Citrate: Calcium citrate is recommended for the maintenance of bones and the prevention of bone loss that may result from malabsorption and decreased intake of foods that contain calcium.

The general recommendation for loss prevention and bone maintenance is 1,000 to 1,500mg of supplemental calcium citrate with vitamin D daily. It is best to divide doses into 500mg or less per serving. Calcium citrate should be in chewable or liquid form.

Iron: Iron deficiency is relatively common in surgical weight loss patients, more so in women than men.

According to Swilley, "Patient risk for iron deficiency is due to the decrease in stomach HCl and decreased intake, and individual risk is associated with heavy menstruation. Symptoms of iron deficiency include anemia, fatigue, hair-loss, feeling cold, pagophagia (significant chewing and eating ice), and decreased immune function." Lab tests for determining iron deficiency should include serum ferritin levels, serum iron, transferring saturation, total iron binding capacity and hemoglobin. Based on lab results iron supplementation therapy should be individually prescribed to the patient and closely monitored to treat deficiency and avoid toxicity. There is not a "one size fits all" supplement therapy in the treatment of iron deficiency.

Magnesium: Magnesium deficiency has not been reported to be associated with gastric surgery. However, its relationship to bone health and mineralization makes it a key ingredient to our overall nutritional wellness. The RDA for men is 350mg and for women 280mg. A safe recommendation for an upper limit of magnesium from supplements is 350mg.

DIETARY MINERALS AND ORGANIC COMPOUNDS

Sodium: In our overall effort for total wellness a reduced sodium diet plays a key role. A diet high in sodium may lead to high blood pressure and those with high blood pressure are more likely to develop heart disease and stroke. According to the American Heart Association (AHA), the average American eats about 2,900 to 4,300mg sodium a day. That is about 1½-teaspoons of salt. Healthy Americans should try to eat less than 2,300mg salt per day or less than a teaspoon of salt. In addition to table salt we find sodium in products that contain monosodium glutamate (MSG), baking soda, baking powder, disodium phosphate, and any compound that has "sodium" or "Na" in its name.

The AHA suggests limiting consumption of the following foods: salted snacks; fish that is frozen, pre-breaded, pre-fried or smoked; also fish that is canned in oil or brine like tuna, sardines or shellfish; ham, bacon, corned beef, luncheon meats, sausages and hot dogs; canned foods and juices containing salt; commercially made main dishes like hash, meat pies and frozen dinners with more than 700mg of sodium per serving; cheeses and buttermilk; seasoned salts, meat tenderizers and MSG; ketchup, mayonnaise, sauces and salad dressings.

After weight loss surgery most of us will be avoiding the foods listed above by the American Heart Association. We learn that the more processed foods are, the less they settle well with us. In turn we prepare for ourselves cleaner foods in which we control the ingredients. To enhance flavor and control sodium we can use fresh herbs, spices, and sauces made from vegetables, fruits, juice, and wine or reduced sodium broth.

In most cases I prefer to not season with salt while cooking opting to use "finishing salt" at the end of meal preparation. During cooking adding salt in free-pour fashion is risky business because we cannot account for the sodium. Over time free-pour salting tends to increase because our taste buds become less sensitive to the taste of salt, so more is required to achieve the salty flavor we enjoy. By minimizing the addition of salt while cooking and seasoning only at the end with finishing salt we maximize our salt tasting pleasure while lowering our sodium intake.

A good seasoning salt will be of coarse grain and blended with herbs and spices for added flavor. There are many quality finishing salt blends available. They prove that less-is-more when it comes to perfecting food while lowering our sodium intake.

The AHA supports the use of products made without added salt and canned vegetables, beans and shellfish that are processed with reduced salt. They suggest fresh lean meats, skinless poultry, fish, egg whites and tuna canned in water.

Sweet Stuff: Sugar, Sugar Substitutes, Sugar Alcohol: A fundamental tenet of the post weight loss surgery diet is to avoid sweet food that is made with sugar, high fructose corn syrup and other sugar byproducts. Some centers give specific recommendations such as no more than 6-8g sugar per meal; others give absolute boundaries: no sugar. Yet sweetness is one of the four specific tastes that taste buds detect (the other three: salty, sour, and bitter). Patients often report cravings for sweet tastes long after surgery. Avoiding sweets is necessary to prevent weight loss stalls, avert weight gain, and in bypass patients, avoid dumping syndrome.

Patients are tempted to use sugar substitutes and products containing sugar alcohol in place of sugar so they may enjoy a taste of sweetness without the consequences of sugar. The following is a summary of sugar substitutes and sugar alcohols and their impact on our nutritional health.

Artificial Sweeteners are calorie free sugar replacements such as saccharine, aspartame, and sucralose (Splenda®). Dr. Andrew Weil, author of "The Healthy Kitchen" is concerned about the use of artificial sweeteners. In his book he states, "In the first place, there is no evidence that they help anyone lose weight, although that is why people use them. Second, most of them taste funny. And, most important, the highly popular ones may be harmful." He cites studies that link Saccharin and aspartamine to health problems.

Dr. Weil recommends sucralose, sold under the brand name Splenda®. He writes, "It tastes better than aspartame and appears safer."

Splenda®. In general nutritionists working with bariatric clients agree Splenda® is an acceptable sweetener for patients when used in moderation. Many recipes can be adjusted to use all Splenda® or a blend of Splenda® and sugar. For baking, using a blend of sugar and Splenda® produces the best results for texture and moistness yet cuts in half the calories and carbohydrates. Using all Splenda® eliminates all sugar calories, however, some consumers say using all Splenda® results in an unpleasant after taste and unappealing texture.

Sweet "sugar free" products made with sugar alcohol are labeled "for diabetic consumption". Unlike artificial sweeteners that contain no calories, sugar alcohol has about half the calories of sugar. Diabetics can have food with sugar alcohol because the body, using only a small amount of insulin, metabolizes it slowly, much more slowly than sugar.

While sugar alcohols are low in calories and slow to convert to glucose, the downside is they usually cause painful gas, bloating and diarrhea. Packages are labeled: "Warning: excessive consumption can cause a laxative effect" for a good reason. Serving size should be noted and never exceeded. Below are sugar alcohols found on prepared food ingredient lists:

Mannitol is found naturally in pineapples, olives, asparagus, sweet potatoes and carrots. It is only 60% as sweet as sugar, so more product is needed to replicate the sweetness of sugar. Mannitol lingers in the intestines and therefore causes bloating and diarrhea

Sorbitol is found naturally in fruits and vegetables. It is manufactured from corn syrup. Sorbitol has only 50% the relative sweetness. of sugar, which means twice as much must be used to deliver a similar amount of sweetness. It has less of a tendency to cause diarrhea compared to mannitol.

Xylitol is also called "wood sugar" and occurs naturally in straw, corncobs, fruit, vegetables, cereals, mushrooms, and some cereals. Xylitol has the same relative sweetness as sugar.

Lactitol has about 30-40% of sugars sweetening power, but its taste and solubility profile resembles sugar so it is often found in sugar-free ice cream, chocolate, hard and soft candies, baked goods, sugar-reduced preserves and chewing gums.

Isomalt is 45–65% as sweet as sugar and does not tend to lose its sweetness or break down during the heating process. Isomalt absorbs little water, so it is often used in hard candies, toffee, cough drops and lollipops.

Maltitol is 75% as sweet as sugar. It is used in sugar-free hard candies, chewing gum, chocolate-flavored desserts, baked goods and ice cream because it gives a creamy texture to foods.

The American Diabetes Association claims that sugar alcohols are acceptable in a moderate amount but should not be eaten in excess. In addition, weight gain has been seen when these products are overeaten. For bariatric patients, the general advice as in all things is to indulge in moderation.

THE FDA'S ROLE IN DIETARY SUPPLEMENT LABELING:

More than once, I must confess, I have left the dietary supplement aisle empty handed having become confused and overwhelmed by the terms and choices offered. What does any of this mean to me? I pondered. The Federal Drug Administration (FDA) oversees and defines the labeling practices for dietary supplements. But they do not approve or test dietary supplements. The following are details provided by the U.S. Food and Drug Administration Consumer Health Information:

The law defines dietary supplements in part as products taken by mouth that contain a "dietary ingredient." Dietary ingredients include vitamins, minerals, amino acids, and herbs or botanicals, as well as other substances that can be used to supplement the diet.

Dietary supplements come in many forms, including tablets, capsules, powders, energy bars, and liquids. The products are available in stores throughout the United States, as well as on the Internet. They are labeled as dietary supplements.

The FDA suggests you consult with a health care professional before using any dietary supplement. (Yet products are available without a prescription.) Many supplements contain ingredients that have strong biological effects, and such products may not be safe in all people.

Federal law does not require dietary supplements to be proven safe to FDA's satisfaction before they are marketed.

For most claims made in the labeling of dietary supplements, the law does not require the manufacturer or seller to prove to FDA's satisfaction that the claim is accurate or truthful before it appears on the product. The following is a sample of the standard disclaimer seen on most products labeled dietary supplement:

*These statements have not been evaluated by the food and Drug Administration. This product is not intended to diagnose, treat, cure, or prevent any disease.

In general, FDA's role with a dietary supplement product begins after the product enters the marketplace. That is usually the agency's first opportunity to take action against a product that presents a significant or unreasonable risk of illness or injury, or that is otherwise adulterated or misbranded.

Once a dietary supplement is on the market, FDA has certain safety monitoring responsibilities. These include monitoring mandatory reporting or serious adverse events by dietary supplement firms and voluntary adverse event reporting by consumers and health care professionals.

Our first line of defense when taking dietary supplements is to communicate with our health care provider and make informed choices.

We then are responsible to follow through with annual laboratory monitoring (blood work) to ensure the prevention of nutritional deficiency that may result from gastric surgery. As we learned from Swilley, "Lifelong preventative actions, such as supplementation, regular follow-up, and thorough patient education are mandatory for accomplishing all the benefits and avoidance of the health risks associated with bariatric surgery."

PHARMACEUTICAL APPETITE SUPPRESSANTS AFTER WLS

In the twenty years since my gastric bypass many things in obesity treatment have changed. In recent years we are seeing more physicians prescribing pharmaceutical therapies to work with the surgical treatment and lifestyle modifications to produce improved weight loss outcomes. In the late 1990's post-WLS patients who later accepted pharmaceuticals in their weight loss program held this information close. Oddly, among patients there was stigmatic judgement of those who added medication to their program. Made to feel weak or frustrated by well-meaning suggestions that they failed surgery WLS patients tended to slink back from the weight loss surgery communities where their own people shamed and bullied. How ridiculous!

See the Appendix for a complete list of pharmaceutical medications for obesity management.

Do we criticize a heart surgery patient for taking pharmaceuticals to prevent stroke or control high blood pressure? Of course not. We understand a heart condition must be managed with a full program that may include surgery, medication, and lifestyle modification. The same should go for the treatment of obesity. And I believe that now, two decades into the new century we are more enlightened and accepting of the fact that obesity is a disease requiring a variety of treatments to support the individual.

As reported by Robert Ziltzer, MD, FAAP in 2013 , appetite suppressants can play a significant role when patients experience a decline in weight loss or begin to regain lost weight. Sympathomimetic medications act to both decrease appetite and increase basal metabolic rate (BMR). The use of appetite suppressants, such as sympathomimetic medications, can offset the effects of the neuropeptides that tend to favor weight gain. Because there is no time at which the risk of regain resolves, long-term use of medications may be required.

When post-bariatric surgery patients do not lose the expected amount of weight, or begin to regain weight, medical therapy can be a useful adjunct to band fills and an alternative to surgical revision. The compensatory decrease in leptin that occurs with weight loss leads to a lowering of the basal metabolic rate and an increase in hunger. Ziltzer notes that while there is controversy regarding a "set point" of one's weight, the tendency to regain is a continuing problem, especially after 3 to 5 years postoperatively. The decrease in leptin remains low for at least one year, and likely much longer. Leptin seems to be a signal that prevents starvation during times of calorie restriction.

Long-term use of appetite suppressants is becoming more widely accepted among obesity medicine specialists. Bariatric Times, the professional journal of the American Society of Metabolic and Bariatric Medicine, recently reviewed USDA-FDA-approved weight loss medications available. A brief summary of the widely used pharmaceuticals is provided in the Appendix. As always, please talk to your doctor about your medication options and use prescription medication as directed.

TAKING MEDICINES - WHAT TO ASK YOUR DOCTOR[1]

Know what medicines, vitamins, and herbal supplements you take.

- Make a list of your medicines to keep in your wallet. Download this wallet card and print form.
- Take time to understand the purpose of your medicine.
- Ask questions when you don't know the meaning of related words, or when instructions aren't clear. And write down the answers to your questions.
- Bring a family member or friend to the pharmacy or to your doctor's visits to help you retain the information you are given.

New Prescriptions. Get information about your new medicine: When your doctor prescribes a medicine, find out about it. Ask questions, such as:

- What is the name of the medicine? Why am I taking this medicine? How long will it take to work?
- What is the name of the condition this medicine will treat?
- How long will it take to work?
- How should I store the medicine? Does it need to be refrigerated?
- Can the pharmacist substitute a cheaper, generic form of the medicine?
- Will the medicine create conflicts with other medicines I take?

Critical User Information. Find out how to take the medicine: Ask your doctor, pharmacist, or nurse about the correct way to take your medicine. Ask questions, such as:

- When and how often should I take the medicine? As needed, or on a schedule?

---

[1] Shared with permission National Institutes of Health (NIH*) U.S. National Library of Medicine

- Do I take medicine before, with, or between meals?
- How long will I have to take it?
- Know what to expect with the new medicine: Ask about how you will feel.
- How will I feel once I start taking this medicine? How will I know if this medicine is working?
- What side effects might I expect? Should I report them?
- Are there any lab tests to check the medicine's level or for any harmful side effects?
- Ask if this new medicine fits in with your other medicines:
- Are there other medicines or activities I should avoid when taking this medicine?
- Will this medicine change how my other medicines work? (Ask about both prescription and over-the-counter medicines.)
- Will this medicine change how any of my herbal or dietary supplements work?
- Ask if your new medicine interferes with eating or drinking:
- Can I drink alcohol when taking this medicine? How much?
- Is it OK to eat or drink food before or after I take the medicine?
- If I forget to take it, what should I do?
- What should I do if I feel I want to stop taking this medicine? Is it safe to just stop?

When to call the doctor or pharmacist:
- You have questions or you are confused or uncertain about the directions for your medicine.
- You are having side effects from the medicine. Do not stop taking the medicine without telling your doctor. You might need a different dose or a different medicine.
- Your medicine looks different than you expected.
- Your refill medicine is different than what you usually get.

144

BODY MASS INDEX

We, as bariatric patients, are intimately familiar with the term Body Mass Index (BMI). Here is a brief review of what it means. There are many reliable BMI calculator apps available for download from your app store. Online you can trust the BMI Calculator at the National Institutes of Health website https://www.nih.gov/ (*U.S. Department of Health and Human Services*).

Body Mass Index is a measure of a person's weight relative to height. A BMI of 25 is the bull's eye: overweight people can aim to lose weight to achieve that target and underweight people can aim to gain weight to near 25 but not exceed it. Well over half of adults in the United States have a BMI greater than 25. It should be noted that BMI reflect height and weight measures and not body composition. To its disadvantage, BMI does not reflect body fat, and it may misclassify very muscular people as overweight.

In the process of our recovery from morbid obesity the BMI is a useful tool in charting progress and keeping tabs on maintenance.

OBESITY MEDICINE PHYSICIAN

Perhaps one of the greatest advances to come from designating obesity a disease is the emergence of the "Obesity Medicine Physician." For years studies have shown that obesity management is only effective when the patient commits to lifelong changes in diet and lifestyle and is supported by a multifaceted process that includes medical, psychosocial, and nutritional and fitness counselling. Yet how many of us have been frustrated with this scenario: "my primary care doctor doesn't understand weight loss surgery; I don't have a nutritionist; I am no longer in contact with my bariatric center; I am all alone in this." Sound familiar?

The American Board of Obesity Medicine (ABOM), chartered in 2011, aims to change this by certifying physicians who have achieved a higher level of competency and understanding in obesity care by completing specialized education. Called diplomates, the board defines the certified "Obesity Medicine Physician" as a "physician with expertise in the sub-specialty of obesity medicine. This sub-specialty requires competency in and a thorough understanding of the treatment of obesity and the genetic, biologic, environmental, social, and behavioral factors that contribute to obesity."

"Patients seeking comprehensive obesity care services are seen by a multidisciplinary team that provides a range of treatments including lifestyle management, pharmacotherapy, and bariatric surgery," said Dr. Robert Kushner, Chair of the ABOM. "Since obesity is viewed as a chronic relapsing disease, patients benefit from the integration of treatment approaches and expertise." Of interest to the WLS community, the ABOM aims to improve the lasting post-surgery care bariatric patients receive. "Postoperative rehabilitation and long-term follow up should include dietary, exercise, and psychological counseling. It is the role of the obesity medicine physician to coordinate the long-term nonsurgical care of the patient."

Physicians who are certified by ABOM are known as Diplomates of the American Board of Obesity Medicine. According to Kushner board certified physicians have demonstrated competency in all aspects of obesity care. "For patients considering bariatric surgery, the obesity specialist leads a team of other healthcare providers, including a registered dietitian, mental healthcare provider, nurse practitioner, or physician assistant in guiding comprehensive preoperative assessment and managing the patient through the perioperative and postoperative experience." This multi-faceted approach significantly improves the patient experience and quality of care they receive.

FIND AN OBESITY MEDICINE PHYSICIAN

If you are interested in finding a certified ABOM obesity medicine physician take advantage of the online physician directory to locate a professional in your area. Go to the ABOM Diplomate Directory Terms of Service page. Once you review the terms click "Accept" and search by name or state. ABOM Diplomate Directory Terms of Service link: http://abom.org/

Obesity Medicine Physician

An obesity medicine physician is a physician with expertise in the sub-specialty of obesity medicine. This sub-specialty requires competency in and a thorough understanding of the treatment of obesity and the genetic, biologic, environmental, social, and behavioral factors that contribute to obesity.

The obesity medicine physician employs therapeutic interventions including diet, physical activity, behavioral change, and pharmacotherapy.

The obesity medicine physician utilizes a comprehensive approach, and may include additional resources such as nutritionists, exercise physiologists, psychologists and bariatric surgeons as indicated to achieve optimal results.

Additionally, the obesity medicine physician maintains competency in providing pre- peri- and post-surgical care of bariatric surgery patients, promotes the prevention of obesity, and advocates for those who suffer from obesity.

WHEN DISASTER STRIKES ARE YOU WLS READY?

As much as we would like to believe our world is safe the fact is emergencies and disasters happen every day. Are you prepared to manage your weight loss surgery special needs in the event of an emergency? Current polling shows that nearly half of American families do not have an emergency plan or an emergency supply kit in the home. When disaster strikes it is too late to plan and prepare. In addition to the standard preparation special care must be given to the needs of the weight loss surgery patient in the event of a crisis. Our 5-Star source for quality emergency preparedness information is the American Red Cross. Please take time to their website for timely emergency preparedness information, worksheets, checklists, and apps. http://www.redcross.org/prepare/disaster

Emergency Preparedness for Weight Loss Surgery Patients

Following weight loss surgery patients make a multitude of adjustments in their lives to accommodate the dietary and nutritional needs of an altered gastric digestive system. Even if weight loss has long been accomplished patients who have undergone gastric bypass, gastric banding or gastric sleeve surgical procedures must, for the rest of their life, maintain rigorous nutritional and dietary habits in order to be healthy. After time these adjustments feel like second nature to the patient and even those around them. But in preparing an emergency kit for use in the wake of a natural or national disaster it is essential that weight loss surgery patients treat themselves as "special needs" and ensure their nutritional and dietary needs are provided for in the event the emergency kit is put into service.

Flood, fire, national disaster, or the loss of power from high winds, snow, or ice frequently jeopardize the health and safety of thousands of Americans each year. Recently weather events and natural disasters have been particularly harsh throughout the world and many thousands have found themselves without food, shelter or warmth. While we cannot prevent natural or national disasters, we can assemble emergency supply kits to improve our survivability when disaster strikes.

A well-prepared basic emergency supply kit will contain items to provide for the basics of survival: fresh water, food, clean air and warmth. The

Federal Emergency Management Agency (FEMA) recommends the following items be included in a basic emergency supply kit:

- o Water, one gallon of water per person per day for a least three days, for drinking and sanitation
- o Food, at least a three-day supply of non-perishable food
- o Battery-powered or hand crank radio and NOAA Weather Radio with tone alert and extra batteries for both
- o Flashlight and extra batteries
- o First aid kit
- o Whistle to signal for help
- o Dust mask, to help filter contaminated air and plastic sheeting and duct tape to shelter-in-place
- o Moist towelettes, garbage bags and plastic ties for personal sanitation
- o Personal hygiene items
- o Tools to turn off utilities and a checklist of how to disable utilities
- o Can opener for food (if kit contains canned food)
- o Local maps
- o Cell phone with chargers
- o Emergency readiness kits should provide water, food, clean air and warmth for 72 hours.
- o The WLS specifics: Keeping that in mind a "special needs" weight loss surgery patient should consider including the following items in their personal readiness kit:
- o Vitamins and supplements for three days. Additional dosages of vitamins B and C may be included to relieve stress and boost immunity.
- o Non-NSAID over-the-counter pain relief medicine. Most surgical weight loss patients are discouraged from using NSAID medication for pain relief. Make sure acceptable OTC pain relief is included in the First aid kit.

149

o   Vitamin fortified or protein fortified powder drink mixes in individual packages. These are useful in adding minerals and nutrients to the diet while stretching the water supply which in a disaster can be limited. When water is vitamin and mineral enhanced it provides hydration with vitamin and mineral nutrition.

o   Ready-to-Drink (RTD) and Ready-to-Eat (RTE) protein drinks and protein bars. A weight loss surgery patient must have a minimum of 60 grams protein per day for best health. Provide at least 60 grams of dietary protein per day for three days of emergency use.

o   Sugar free hard candy to supplement food intake and keep the mouth moist.

o   Additional bedding or clothing for warmth. Body temperature regulation is difficult for those having lost body weight or body mass. Provide extra items for warmth in the event of a disaster that subjects the weight loss surgery patient to extreme cold or elements.

Emergency response information for the treatment of a bariatric patient including contact numbers. Make this information readily available to first responders. Gather items for the emergency preparedness kit in one location. Stow the items in a portable duffel bag or plastic bin that is accessible and labeled for easy access in the event of an emergency. Ideally each household member will have a kit tailored for their needs. Periodically check the kit and replenish items that have expired. Make certain all contact information is current. It is not easy to think about facing a disaster, but should the day come when the emergency kit is needed a little preparation will be of good use.

EMERGENCY FIRST AID FOR DUMPING SYNDROME

We have discussed the cause of dumping syndrome earlier. When a dumping situation occurs first aid measures should be taken to relieve some of the distress and discomfort associated with the insulin crisis.

Recognize the crisis. The symptoms of dumping syndrome will manifest immediately after eating or within three hours of eating. Each person is unique in the gastric dumping response; however, the common symptoms may include nausea, vomiting, bloating, cramping, diarrhea, profuse sweating followed by chills, dizziness and fatigue. When insulin levels return to normal symptoms subside.

Provide for Physical Comfort: At the onset of a dumping episode the patient may first notice a sense of disorientation or confusion. This indicates the body is beginning to panic over an excess of insulin flooding the bloodstream. One who has suffered from dumping previously will probably feel a sense of despair as they realize the onset of dumping syndrome. Providing for physical comfort is the first response to a dumping episode. Efforts to interrupt or halt the dumping episode are futile. Many patients of gastric bypass familiar with dumping prefer to isolate from others finding a cool place in which to lie down. Symptoms may include vomiting or diarrhea so patients should find a restful place near a bathroom. Many will experience a short period of profuse sweating followed by a longer period of chills: providing a blanket is useful to relieve chills. A patient will reach for the blanket when it is needed, the caregiver should not attempt to cover the patient unless asked to do so. The patient may experience symptoms of sensory disorder including extreme and abnormal sensitivity light, sound, and touch. These are transient symptoms and many patients find relief when lights are dimmed, and they are resting in a reduced-noise environment. Many patients say they prefer not to be comforted by touch from their caregiver because of acute sensitivity to touch during the dumping event.

Hydration and Electrolyte Beverages: Gastric bypass patients who are suffering from dumping syndrome may have been mildly dehydrated prior to the dumping episode. It is important to return the body to a hydrated state by sipping room temperature water or electrolyte fortified sports beverages. Patients should be discouraged from partaking of sugar sweetened beverages or juice to correct the insulin imbalance. The body is already in a reactionary and corrective state to the insulin surge and efforts to speed-up the correction process seldom accelerate balance.

When to Seek Emergency Care: Patients should seek emergency medical care when the symptoms of dumping syndrome last for an extended period. If a patient loses consciousness immediately seek emergency medical care and provide details for the patient including the bariatric procedure, history of diabetes or hypoglycemia, and an account of food intake prior to the dumping episode.

Not all weight loss surgery patients experience dumping syndrome. It most commonly occurs in patients of malabsorptive procedures, specifically gastric bypass. Patients of adjustable gastric banding (lap-band) and gastric sleeve are not known to have dumping syndrome. Following an episode of dumping patients should consult their bariatric center to identify the cause of the event and plan to avoid episodes in the future.

IT'S NOT YOUR FAULT: REVISIONS HAPPEN

I continue to be surprised, after all we have been through regarding our obesity and recovery, that when it comes time to discuss the possibility of a revision procedure, we are timid, embarrassed, ashamed and hush-hush about it. Somehow, we think when something goes wrong it is our fault and one more time we are a failure. Consider this: if your dear friend who was enjoying remission from cancer suddenly learned the disease had returned would you lay blame on her? Would you cause her to feel shame? Then why, when our disease fights back, do we blame ourselves?

As the medical journals define them "bariatric revisions are performed on failed gastric bypass not on failed patients." And often the failure of the original surgery has more to do with the experience and skill of the surgeon than the ability of the patient to use the tool effectively. In fact, Bariatric Times, the professional journal for Bariatric medicine, says the surgeon's learning curve for laparoscopic gastric bypass is one of the longest surgical learning curves and improperly performed procedures result in the operation failing the patient from the beginning. (It should be noted surgical failures are seldom reported in banding procedures due to constant monitoring and adjustment of the bands.)

The Roux-en-Y gastric bypass (RYGB) is the most commonly performed bariatric procedure in the United States and Bariatric Times reports a long-term failure rate of 20 to 35 percent. According to those statistics 20 to 35 percent of patients never achieve expected weight loss and many regain significant weight following excess weight loss.

If you are thinking, "That's me" then here is what you can do. First, I strongly encourage you to give the 5 Day Pouch Test a try. (You knew I was going to say that, right?) What do you have to lose? Give yourself a chance to turn things around. A real honest-to-goodness sincere try at making it work for you. At the end of the 5 days consider how you feel mentally and physically. Do you have new faith in your gastric surgery, or do you feel your surgery has failed you?

I trust you to know your body better than anyone else. If your surgery has failed, seek consult with a surgical center that specializes in gastric revision surgery. Make an appointment and provide, if possible, your original operative report to the physician. Make notes and be prepared to answer honestly a nutritional evaluation that will include questions about your snacking, grazing and volume eating habits. The only way a revision procedure will be helpful to you is if you are completely honest answering these questions. Be prepared, with notes. If possible, provide a timeline of your weight loss and weight gain following your original bariatric procedure. As part of your evaluation you will undergo anatomic testing which may include both upper endoscopy and upper gastrointestinal (GI) contrast studies, as they are complementary in the evaluation of anatomy and cause of weight gain after bariatric surgery. Endoscopy provides useful information about the pouch and stoma while upper GI detects esophageal and Roux limb abnormalities.

Using the data collected in your nutritional and anatomic evaluation a treatment plan will be made that may include a revision procedure. The two most common bariatric revisions are the Restorative Obesity Surgery, Endolumenal (ROSE) and the StomaphyX: both minimally invasive.

Restorative Obesity Surgery, Endolumenal (Rose): The ROSE procedure is performed using a four-channel tube and surgical tools that do not require an incision. The patient is anesthetized and the channel tube is inserted through the patient's mouth into the stomach pouch. Surgical tools are maneuvered through the channels and folds are made in the tissue around the stoma to decrease the size. Anchors are then placed in the stomach pouch to reduce its volume. Patients who are treated in the morning are usually released from the hospital in the afternoon. Few patients report discomfort from the procedure with the most common complaint being short-term sore throat from the instruments. This is a relatively new procedure and long-term data are not yet available.

Recovery is quick and patients generally return to normal activity within a matter of days. As always, follow the specific guidelines prescribed by the surgeon providing your care.

StomaphyX: This is a non-invasive procedure in which surgical instruments are inserted through the mouth into the stomach pouch. The patient is anesthetized during this procedure, which is frequently performed on an outpatient basis. The surgeon reduces the size of the stoma or stomach outlet by partially closing it with sutures. "A stoma that has dilated to greater than 2cm is considered ineffective for weight loss or weight maintenance and is considered a surgical failure causing weight regain," according to Parikh and Bessler in Bariatric Times.

The StomaphyX procedure does not require abdominal or internal surgical incisions, it preserves future treatment options, it is essentially painless, recovery is rapid, and it may be customized for unique procedures for different anatomies.

Banding over Bypass: A final revision strategy sometimes practiced is placing a laparoscopic adjustable gastric band (LapBand or Realize band) over an existing gastric bypass. The intent is to recreate the satiety that gastric bypass patients experienced early after the initial surgery. The addition of the band allows frequent adjustments in the long-term management of weight loss and weight maintenance.

Do what is right for you: That is a brief overview of the current practices in gastric surgery revision. There is no finger pointing, no laying blame, no standing in the corner of shame. Revisions happen. When a revision is the appropriate protocol seek qualified medical care with the skill and experience to treat your case professionally and appropriately.

CHAPTER 6: DAILY INTELLIGENT EATING TRIUMPHS

Now that we have reviewed emotional, dietary, and factual information of our weight loss surgery experience it is time to put it all together for our Day 6 success. This is where Day 6 becomes at once and forever the DAY 6 DIET:

After reading this far you know that the DAY 6 DIET is liberating, not confining. You know that following guidelines gives you the choice and opportunity to treat yourself well with good nutrition and intelligent choices every day. You know a well-thought plan will spare you the anguish of poor choices and the unavoidable self-loathing that follows. Nobody goes into weight loss surgery hoping for only a year or two of good results: we want to revel in good health for the rest of our lives. Nobody wants to suffer the disappointment, frustration and embarrassment of weight regain. We do not want to return to suffering the comorbidities of obesity. If I have heard it once I have heard it one-thousand times ten, "Weight loss surgery was my last hope; my final solution."

I declared it my final decision in 1999. When did you declare it yours?

The DAY 6 DIET is a kind-hearted, reasonable, capable and intelligent method of dietary and health management making the most of our surgical weight loss tool. We brought our tool back into the very world in which we became fat armed with Four Rules and a heart full of hope. We knew, by memorization, what we had to do to get through the first weeks and months following surgery. But after that the instructions become vague and we found ourselves wandering, possibly feeling alone. The Four Rules are not enough. They don't address emotional or social issues; they barely give a nod to the physiological issues. And they don't explain well enough why we need to eat protein first or avoid slider foods or why alcohol affects us so differently.

We are intelligent people: A little more information would have served us well and perhaps helped us avoid some of the struggles. But all is not lost. After doing the 5 Day Pouch Test (if we were off track and stuck in a slider food habit) we have reset ourselves to a newbie-like feeling and here we are at Day 6. We can begin Day 6 with our new knowledge and embrace the DAY 6 DIET.

The DAY 6 DIET is what I wish I had been counseled to follow in the first place. And with all humility, I am confident if I had been, I would still be following the tenets of it today. I know this because I have been living the DAY 6 DIET for the last several years since I figured it out on my own.

I believe by now that even those most jaded to the word "diet" will agree DAY 6 DIET is a concept they can embrace. It simply means that we chose daily to make intelligent choices about food; our daily provisions. We have a skeleton plan. We understand the terms of our weight loss surgery: we agreed to them at the time of surgery and surrendering to them is freedom. A consequence of that surrender is independence from obesity; improved health; and emotional freedom from self-loathing. A plan allows us to affect weight loss and accomplish weight maintenance. A plan allows us error and forgiveness: when eggs are broken, we clean them up and move forward. A plan provides coping strategies: we Stay on PAR and we practice retreat with DDA: Distance & Distraction Action. We respect and respond to our Needful Pings with Four First: Oxygen, Hydration, Wiggle Therapy, and Rest. We seek support, understanding and commiseration from our peers. We do not walk alone.

We use knowledge so that we understand what is happening to our bodies and why. We do not relinquish our health to fate because experience has taught us fate is not always on our side.

We take ownership of our medical care being informed patients asking well-thought questions. We document weights and measurements serving as our own personal statisticians. We provide honest and detailed health histories to our medical team so they can best serve us. When medical complications, such as a revision, occur, we seek understanding and healing. We do not place blame.

I have been asked, "Why Day 6? Why no Day 7 or Day 8?"

The answer is simple: Day 6 works. Nothing about Day 6 needs to be done differently on the following day or the following day and so forth. Planning, predictability, consistency all aggregates in our favor to accomplish the goals of weight loss, weight maintenance, good health, and balanced emotional and mental wellness.

While I hesitate to make a religious tie to a dietary lifestyle, it should be noted that in the traditional Christian theory of creationism based on the Book of Genesis in the Holy Bible, it was on the 6th day that the Lord commands the land to bring forth living creatures: wild beasts, livestock, reptiles. He then creates man and woman in His "image" and "likeness". The Lord gives the animals and man plants to eat and he calls the creation "very good." It was on the seventh day the Lord rested.

Who wouldn't want to repeat Day 6?

Not long ago an old man wearing thick horn-rimmed glasses, walking a bit bent carrying a heavy box, came to our home to make a repair. Upon the floor he placed a canvas cloth. I watched as he opened the heavy box and one-by-one removed each tool from within. Without speaking he placed the tools upon the cloth in an order that only he understood.

When he stood and opened the piano lid to begin tuning the neglected instrument the box was empty of tools. The old man was ready to engage fully the task of making beautiful the instrument knowing exactly where each tool was for any purpose it might be needed. The old man spent many hours tinkering with the out-of-tune piano. He never abandoned it, as I was afraid he might, saying it was too far-gone and beyond repair.

As the sun was setting, one by one, he returned each tool to its proper place in the box. "It is good," he told me patting the old piano as if it were a wise old dog on the mend. He took the heavy box and carried it away. I played the piano: it never sounded so sweet.

Following is the DAY 6 DIET Daily Checklist. It is divided into four categories: nutritional, physical, emotional & spiritual, and social wellness. This is your canvas cloth upon which your tools are laid as you begin the task of tuning your body on every Day 6. Like the piano tuner, before you take on the task of the day, you lay out your tools in preparation. When you need that tool, you reach for it and use it with skill and finesse. And at the end of the day you can put your tools back in place and say, "It is good." Tomorrow it starts anew: Day 6.

When we begin the journey of weight loss surgery there is a sense that it is mostly of the body: the food we eat and the exercise in which we engage. But as time goes forward we observe it is as much about our emotional, spiritual and social health as anything else. The checklist covers these areas so that as a whole being we may traverse the obstacles of Day 6 using our tools to do our best and tune our instrument.

In the next part of this book, Cooking with Kaye, you will learn weekly menu planning. Use this tool with your daily checklist.

As you travel though life you will gather more coping tools for your daily success with weight loss surgery. Add them to your toolbox and share them with your fellow travelers on this path. The journey need never be lonely again.

DAY 6 DIET DAILY CHECKLIST

Did I nurture my nutritional health today?

Protein First (60-105g Protein)

Lots of Water – 64+ ounces: Liquid Restrictions

No Snacking: avoided Slider Foods

Vitamin & mineral supplements?

Was I mindful of my fork?

Did I make intelligent food choices?

Did I nurture my physical health today?

30 minutes of exercise

Wiggle therapy

Breathing exercises

Did I nurture my emotional & spiritual health today?

Was I my own caregiver today?

Did I stay on PAR?

Have I reinvented Head Hunger?

Did I clean up and forgive my dropped eggs?

Did I practice receptiveness to new things?

Have I expressed appreciation?

Am I making progress: raking my rocks.?

Did I nurture my social wellness today?

Did I seek support when I needed it?

Did I offer support to those whom I could help?

Did I make a silly memory with someone I cherish today?

Did I practice Distance & Distraction when retreat was necessary?

Summary:

Tomorrow:

DAY 6 DIET DAILY CHECKLIST

Did I nurture my nutritional health today?

Protein First (60-105g Protein)

Lots of Water – 64+ ounces: Liquid Restrictions

No Snacking: avoided Slider Foods

Vitamin & mineral supplements?

Was I mindful of my fork?

Did I make intelligent food choices?

Did I nurture my physical health today?

30 minutes of exercise

Wiggle therapy

Breathing exercises

Did I nurture my emotional & spiritual health today?

Was I my own caregiver today?

Did I stay on PAR?

Have I reinvented Head Hunger?

Did I clean up and forgive my dropped eggs?

Did I practice receptiveness to new things?

Have I expressed appreciation?

Am I making progress: raking my rocks.?

Did I nurture my social wellness today?

Did I seek support when I needed it?

Did I offer support to those whom I could help?

Did I make a silly memory with someone I cherish today?

Did I practice Distance & Distraction when retreat was necessary?

Summary:

Tomorrow:

Download the Day 6 free worksheets at 5DayPouchTest.com > DOWNLOADS.

PART III: COOKING WITH KAYE

I did not know how much I love to cook until several years after weight loss surgery. Prior to weight loss surgery all I knew is that I loved to eat. Surgery changes the way we eat and for me, function followed form. I needed to learn how to pack a whole lot of protein and nutrition in a little package to get the most bang for my bite. I have learned a great deal about what I like to eat, what sets well with my stomach pouch, and what serves a family of normal eaters well as they enjoy a meal alongside my little plate and me.

It is my pleasure to share with you some of our family favorites that we have enjoyed the last several years. For the best results and wonderfully satisfying meals pay close attention to your ingredients. Look for the freshest fish on ice at the market. Fresh meat and poultry yield savory goodness. Find the brightest ripest fruit at the farm stand. Buy the food grown closest to your home. Pick the ripe tomato from your own vine. When you begin with terrific ingredients you have done the right thing. You have triumphed. And that is what makes the DAY 6 DIET a way of life. Daily Intelligent Eating Triumphs.

Use these Cooking with Kaye recipes as your launching pad to culinary discovery. It will not hurt my feelings at all if you change up a recipe to suit your taste or needs. In fact, drop me a note and let me know how you took some of my recipes and made them work for you. Remember, we are all in this together and I enjoy learning from you.

Important Note: Serving Size: For purposes of continuity recipe serving size and nutrient values are calculated and measured on the Daily Values standard for a 2,000 calorie/day diet for adults, developed by the Food and Drug Administration (FDA). It is understood that people who have undergone a restrictive bariatric surgical procedure will eat less than the standard serving size, and that people with different bariatric procedures will eat different volumes of food per serving. Please use the serving size and nutrient values provided as the baseline factor from which to calculate and adjust your specific and unique dietary intake.

Please visit my author's page on Amazon.com for a current catalog of recipe books and lifestyle books to support your on-going efforts at weight management with WLS. https://www.amazon.com/-/e/B00LWITO8I

Day 6 Menu Planning Strategy

We have established that mindful planning surpasses any other action we can take to avoid leaving our nutritional fate to chance. Over the years I have learned that what foils our good intentions to have a plan is the method: too complicated, too time consuming, too detailed, too boring, or too rigid. Check any of the above.

We entered weight loss surgery knowing the commitment was for life, so we need a plan that fits into our life: we do not need to fit our life into the plan. Just like we are learning to own our surgical tool our way, we must own our planning tool the same way.

Begin your menu planning by noting meals you will prepare and plan for those days. Note on your calendar meal engagements and take advantage of the Day 6 strategies to plan your approach for meals away from home. Next, plan your protein main dishes: go for a minimum 21 grams of protein per meal. Look for opportunities to double-up on ingredients or cook once-eat twice meals. Most evening meals can become tomorrow's lunch with happy results. Meal planning is a good time to:

- Try new recipes and ingredients
- Experiment with different preparation and cooking methods
- Compose your grocery list as you plan meals
- Be prepared for a change of plans
- Strive to improve your menu planning skills each week

Be sure to check-out our new weight loss surgery specific planners. Find them on Amazon (Kaye Bailey page: https://www.amazon.com/-/e/B00LWITO8I) and enjoy a tool to make meal planning a breeze.

The recipes in this book have been tested for their nutritional value and taste appeal. I have learned that if it tastes good there is a great sense of satisfaction and Day 6 never feels like dieting purgatory. That is why we can call it the DAY 6 DIET and that is why it is easy to make intelligent choices and triumph. Once I learned that I could love food, just love it a different way, an entirely new and enlightening adventure awaited.

Food plays a key role in our social dynamics and if, because of surgical weight loss, we suffer the loss of that dynamic we lose much. The gathering at the table is more about a place of communion for life's large and small events: small Sunday suppers and grand holiday extravaganzas. It is about bonding and fellowship in a setting-the table- that is familiar and uncomplicated.

Art Smith in his beautiful work, "Back to the Table" writes, "Getting back to the table allows us to love and nurture each other and renew connections to our families-however they may be configured in this diverse and ever-changing society. Such connections are crucial in a fast-paced world where we feel more disconnected every day. One of the best ways I know to restore that daily balance is to sit down at the table." I wish you blessings on your table and hope that some of these recipes are served there.

WEEK OF:

MONDAY

TUESDAY

WEDNESDAY

THURSDAY

FRIDAY

SATURDAY

SUNDAY

SHOPPING LIST:

WEEK OF: MEAL PLANNER

MONDAY

TUESDAY

WEDNESDAY

THURSDAY

FRIDAY

SATURDAY

SUNDAY

SHOPPING LIST:

Download the Day 6 free worksheets at 5DayPouchTest.com > DOWNLOADS.

Tonics, Shakes & Smoothies

Liquid refreshment plays a key role in our post-surgical weight loss diet. In fact, in the early days and weeks following surgery we live on liquids, mostly clear broths and protein enhanced beverages. It is my personal preference to make shakes and smoothies an occasional menu selection rather than a daily meal. Here are some of the shakes and smoothies I enjoy as infrequent treats. Most are fruit or vegetable based and they do a stellar job of beating the carb monster cravings.

Smoothie – *noun*: A cold, non-alcoholic beverage typically consisting of blended fruit juice, fruit pulp, flavoring such as cinnamon or vanilla, and milk, mixed with yogurt and/or ice cream. Ice cubes may also be added to provide an ingredient that adds texture and cooling effects. Smoothies are often promoted as nutritional drinks made with low-fat ingredients that contain a variety of vitamins and minerals.

Lemon & Ginger Tonic

This easy-to-make tonic is a cleanser and a stomach soother. It may be used daily or in digestive emergencies. Start the 5 Day Pouch Test with it and continue Day 6 and Beyond with it. It is an ancient remedy for what ails your tummy.

The tonic works because lemon is an astringent that helps remove toxins from our bodies and we soon feel energetic and cleansed. Lemons, limes, oranges, and grapefruits are all antioxidant rich. And they are low-glycemic. That means they won't disrupt our high-protein diet with a sugar surge. We all know that citrus is rich in vitamin C. Vitamin C is a powerful antioxidant with properties that protect both the cells and the blood from free radical damage. Vitamin C helps restore and regenerate the cells. Adequate intake of Vitamin C can decrease the incidence of colds and infection. It improves the skin, hair and nails.

Ingredients:
2 lemons, washed and sliced ½-inch thick
1/2 teaspoon freshly grated ginger*
3 cups boiling water
Honey or artificial sweetener to taste

In a teapot or saucepot combine lemon slices, grated ginger and boiling water. Cover and let steep 10 minutes. Pour tonic through strainer to remove solids. Drink warm adding honey or sweetener to taste. Garnish with lemon slices if desired. Be sure to drink all three cups. This is best first thing in the morning before eating or drinking anything else.

*Ready-to-use ginger is available bottled in the produce section. It is finely minced and prepared with vinegar which is also a digestive aid. For me this handy condiment is as effective as freshly grated ginger and I am more likely to make a tonic when the effort is minimal. This is also an economical option due to the extended shelf life of prepared ginger versus the fresh ginger.

BLACKBERRY-BANANA SMOOTHIE

To increase the protein of this smoothie, add 1 scoop of whey protein powder.

Ingredients:
2 cups soymilk
1 banana, frozen, sliced
1 1/2 cups blackberries, fresh or frozen
1 scoop protein powder

Place all ingredients in blender and process until smooth and creamy. Serve immediately.

Serves 2. Per serving: 241 Calories; 5g Fat; 18g Protein; 32g Carbohydrate; 10g Dietary Fiber.

BLUSHING PEACH ALMOND SMOOTHIE

This is a brunch-worthy smoothie that is particularly lovely served in wine goblets. Peaches are a rich source of beta-carotene, which helps protect the skin from harmful UV sunrays.

Ingredients:
1 cup soymilk
2 large peaches, fresh, peeled, pitted, diced
1 teaspoon vanilla extract
1/2 teaspoon almond extract
1 scoop protein powder
6 ice cubes

Pour the milk into a blender and add the peaches, vanilla, and almond extracts and top with ice. Blend on high speed until smooth. Serve immediately in chilled glasses. Frozen peaches without added syrup will work during the off-season.

Serves 2. Per serving: 140 Calories; 2g Fat; 14g Protein; 14g Carbohydrate; 4g Dietary Fiber.

CARDAMOM LASSI

Health promoting beverages such as our modern smoothies have a long culinary history. The lassi in the Punjab region of India and usually includes yogurt with water or ice and spices. This Lassi is made of yogurt and flavored with lemon, almonds and cardamom. It is not your average food court beverage. I think you'll like it. If you prefer, use nutmeg in place of the cardamom.

Ingredients:
1 quart plain low-fat yogurt
1/4 cup blanched almonds
2 Tablespoons lemon juice
2 packets artificial sweetener
2 teaspoons honey
1 pinch cardamom
1/2 cup ice cubes

Combine all ingredients in blender and blend until smooth and frothy. Taste for sweetness and flavor; add more sugar substitute and cardamom as desired.

Serves 4. Per serving: 221 Calories; 9g Fat; 15g Protein; 23g Carbohydrate; 1g Dietary Fiber.

PAPAYA DREAMSICLE

3/4 cup vanilla soymilk
1 small papaya, peeled, seeded, cut into chunks and frozen
1 ½-teaspoons freshly grated orange peel
1 teaspoon pure vanilla extract
1 scoop protein powder, optional

Place all ingredients in the blender and blend on high speed until smooth. Serve immediately.

Serves 1. Per Serving: 132 Calories; 6g Protein; 4g Fat; 19g Carbohydrate; 5g Dietary Fiber.

COCONUT BANANA SMOOTHIE

Coconut oil has been shown to promote healthy thyroid function and reduce sugar cravings.

Ingredients:
3/4 cup soymilk
1 medium banana, peeled and chunked
1 Tablespoon coconut oil
1 Tablespoon flax seeds, ground
1 teaspoon vanilla extract
6 ice cubes
1 scoop protein powder, unflavored

Pour the milk into a blender and add the banana, coconut oil, flaxseed, and vanilla extract. Blend the mixture until smooth. Then add the ice and blend again until smooth. Serve well chilled.

Serves 2. Per serving: 223 Calories; 10g Fat; 14g Protein;18g Carbohydrate; 4g Dietary Fiber.

STRAWBERRY COCONUT CRÈME

This smoothie is rich in antioxidants and dietary fiber and is an outstanding pre-workout energy booster. If you just cannot stand tofu replace it with plain low-fat yogurt.

Ingredients:
1/2 cup soymilk
5 ounces tofu, soft, silken
1/3 cup coconut, grated
1 teaspoon vanilla extract
8 medium strawberries, fresh or frozen, no sugar added
3 medium dates
6 ice cubes
1 scoop protein powder, unflavored

Pour the milk into a blender and add the tofu, coconut, vanilla, strawberries, dates, ice cubes, and protein powder. Blend on high speed until smooth. Serve immediately.

Serves 2. Per serving: 226 Calories; 9g Fat; 18g Protein; 18g Carbohydrate; 5g Dietary Fiber.

SAVORY SQUASH SMOOTHIE

This is a cold savory soup smoothie that is nearly as effective as grandma's chicken soup in boosting health and recovery during cold and flu season. I prefer to warm it gently, but it is quite tasty as a cold soup sipped from a glass. This is a great way to use leftover cooked squash. Canned pumpkin may be substituted for the squash.

Ingredients:
1 cup onion, chopped
2 cloves garlic
1 teaspoon olive oil
1/2 cup evaporated milk
1 cup butternut squash, cooked and mashed
1/2 cup yogurt, low-fat
1 scoop protein powder, chicken flavored

1 teaspoon ground cinnamon
1/4 teaspoon ground cloves
1 cup chicken broth, reduced sodium

Over medium heat in a small skillet cook and stir the onion and garlic in the olive oil for about 10 minutes or until the onion is transparent. Pour the milk into the blender and add the onion mixture, squash, yogurt, protein powder, cinnamon, cloves, and chicken broth. Blend on high speed until smooth. Serve chilled.

Serves 4. Per serving: 136 Calories; 5g Fat; 10g Protein; 13g Carbohydrate; 2g Dietary Fiber.

Note: Winter Squash have thick skin, a hollow inner cavity containing hard seeds, and dense flesh requiring a longer cooking time than summer squash. The skin on winter squash is not edible and the squash must be cooked before eaten. They are picked when fully ripe, unlike summer squash that are picked before fully ripe. Winter squash are drier and have a sweeter taste than summer squash.

TOMATO LEMON TWIST SMOOTHIE

Tomatoes and lemon are rich in vitamin C and flavonoids that help fight free radicals and boost the immune system. Even though we supplement with vitamin C it is helpful to include fruit and vegetables in our diet that are rich in vitamin C for extra immunity. This smoothie is low carbohydrate and comes together quickly in the blender.

Ingredients:
2 tomatoes, cut into chunks and frozen
1 cup tomato juice, no sodium added
½-lemon, juiced
1 teaspoon grated lemon rind
6 fresh basil leaves, rinsed

Place frozen tomato chunks in the blender with the tomato juice, lemon juice, lemon peel and basil. Blend on high speed until smooth. Serve immediately.

Serves 2. Per serving: 40 Calories; 3g Fat; 2g Protein; 11g Carbohydrate; trace Dietary Fiber.

GREEN TEA PEAR SMOOTHIE

Green tea is thought to facilitate weight loss and have cancer-preventative properties. In Japan there is strong supporting evidence that regular green-tea drinkers have dramatically lower rates of stomach cancer. Use leftover green tea to make the green tea ice cubes used for this delicious and refreshing low-calorie smoothie.

Ingredients:
6 green tea ice cubes
1 cup white grape juice, naturally sweetened
1 medium pear, washed, peeled, cored and cut into chunks

Place all ingredients in blender and blend until smooth. Enjoy immediately.

Serves 2. Per serving: 74 Calories; 2g Fat; 1g Protein; 18g Carbohydrate; trace Dietary Fiber.

EGGS

Most WLS people that I speak with say that eggs play a major role in their diet, and they become fatigued by the same egg recipes day after day. I understand. It is so easy to reach for my old standby, the hard-cooked egg, no guesswork involved.

Eggs play a leading role in our diet because they are a near-perfect source of protein. In fact, they are the standard by which all protein is measured. According to the American Egg Board, "One egg provides 6 grams of protein, or 12% of the Recommended Daily Value. Eggs provide the highest quality protein found in any food because they contain all of the essential amino acids our bodies need in a near-perfect pattern."

More importantly, for us, the high-quality protein found in eggs helps us stay full longer and researchers believe it helps us maintain weight because we are satiated to the point where we refrain from snacking. The AEB reports, "Research shows that eggs eaten at the start of the day can reduce daily calorie intake, prevent snacking between meals and keep you satisfied on those busy days when mealtime is delayed."

Here I have included a variety of my favorite egg recipes from the simply sublime Quick Coffee Cup Scramble to elegant omelets and a delicious and different Scandinavian Country-Style Scramble that I know you will enjoy.

But don't relinquish the good old standby hard cooked egg forever. Sometimes simple is best. Enjoy your eggs!

Perfect Protein: One large egg contains 75 Calories; 6g Protein; 5g Fat; 213mg Cholesterol and 63mg Sodium.

At the market look for Medium, Large, and Extra-large eggs. The recipes in this book have been developed with Large eggs. Buy eggs only in stores where they are kept refrigerated. Check the freshness date, and then open the carton to see if the shells are intact. Do not purchase cartons with broken eggs. Store refrigerated, in the carton and use before the expiration date.

HARD COOKED EGGS

"Research shows that eating high-quality protein foods for breakfast, like eggs, can help you feel more satisfied and energized throughout the day. Make a batch of hard-boiled eggs so you'll have an all-natural, high-quality protein on-the-go meal or snack ready for the busy week ahead." American Egg Board. Visit http://www.incredibleegg.org

Method: Hard Cooked Eggs As instructed by the American Egg Board: Place as many eggs as desired in a single layer in a saucepan. Add enough water to come at least 1 inch above the eggs. Cover saucepan and place on high heat and bring water to a boil. As soon as the water begins to boil turn off heat and remove saucepan from stove. Keep the saucepan covered and let eggs sit in the hot water for 12 to 15-minutes. When time is up run cold water over eggs to cool them. To remove shell, crackle it by tapping gently all over. Roll egg between hands to loosen shell. Peel the eggs starting at the large end. Hold egg under running cold water or dip in bowl of water to help ease off shell. Once they are cooled store hard cooked eggs (in the shell) in the refrigerator, separated from raw eggs, and use within one week of cooking.

Note: Sometimes hard cooked eggs are card "hard boiled eggs". The food industry in recent years has shied away from this description in favor of hard cooked eggs to better describe the approved cooking method described above. Shell eggs that are overcooked in boiling water tend to be rubbery and unpleasant. The above cooking method produces a firm yet tender egg white and firm yet moist egg yolk that is safe to eat and pleasing to the palate.

Egg Cookers: At our house we prepare hard cooked eggs in an electric egg cooker, a small counter-top appliance that uses steam to cook the eggs. The process is straightforward, takes under 10 minutes, and requires no tending. Egg cookers can be found with small kitchen appliances and can cost from $20 to $60 depending upon brand and options.

PICNIC EGGS

Some people call them "stuffed eggs" and others call them "Deviled eggs". I call them picnic eggs. It doesn't matter what you call them, hard cooked eggs with the yolks mashed and seasoned are just plain good and smart food for bariatric patients. One serving (2 stuffed halves) is 6 grams protein and fits perfectly in the pouch. Stuffed eggs are one of those recipes that are family famous: you know, Aunt Hazel's Famous Picnic Eggs or Uncle Gino's World-Famous Deviled eggs. Here are a few of my "famous" Picnic Eggs.

Basic Ingredients:
6 hard-cooked eggs
1/4 cup mayonnaise
¼-teaspoon salt
Paprika, for garnish

Basic Picnic Eggs: Slice eggs in half lengthwise. Gently remove yolks and place in small bowl; with fork, finely mash yolks. Stir in mayonnaise and salt until smooth. With spoon, pile yolk mixture into egg white halves. Cover and refrigerate.

Delicious variations:

- ○ **Bacon-Stuffed Eggs**: Add 2 to 3 tablespoons crumbled, crisp, cooked bacon to yolk mixture. Garnish with paprika.
- ○ **Radish-Stuffed Eggs**: Add 3 tablespoons minced radishes to yolk mixture. Garnish with radish half-moon slices.

- o **Green Stuffed Eggs**: Add 1 mashed avocado to yolk mixture. Garnish with chopped fresh parsley.
- o **Olive-Stuffed Eggs**: Mince 6 black olives: use to garnish basic picnic eggs.
- o **Mustard-Stuffed Eggs**: Add 1 teaspoon Dijon-style mustard and 1/4 teaspoon dry mustard to yolk mixture. Garnish with freshly ground black pepper.

Serves 6: 2 stuffed egg halves per serving. Average nutrients per serving: 143 Calories; 13g Fat; 6g Protein; 1g Carbohydrate; 0g Dietary Fiber.

Fun Fact! *Did you know that egg yolk is an excellent source of healthy monosaturated and polyunsaturated fats and almost half of the high-quality protein found in eggs?*

SHRIMP AND EGG SALAD ON BUTTERHEAD LETTUCE

Authentic Dijon mustard originates in France and is labeled as such, much as Champagne is only authentic if the sparkling wine originates in the Champagne region of France. Dijon-style mustard is any grainy style mustard. There are many great gourmet varieties of mustard available on the market today and experimenting with them is an inexpensive and delectable method to bring variety to routine dishes such as egg salad.

Ingredients:
1 head butterhead lettuce, rinsed and drained
4 eggs, hard-cooked, chopped
3 Tablespoons low-fat mayonnaise
2 Tablespoons Dijon-style mustard
½-teaspoon celery salt
1 teaspoon dried onion, minced
4 ounces bay shrimp, cooked
Paprika, for garnish
Parsley sprigs, for garnish

Carefully remove the leaves from the lettuce keeping them in cup shape. Place them on a platter and cover with a slightly damp paper towel. Refrigerate to keep them crisp while making the egg salad.

Mix together the chopped eggs, mayonnaise, Dijon-style mustard, celery salt and minced dried onion. Cover and chill until just before serving. (Mixture may be stored up to 6 hours before serving).

To Assemble: Place one lettuce cup on each of four chilled salad plates. Place 1/4 of the egg salad in each lettuce cup and top each with one ounce of bay shrimp. Sprinkle with paprika and garnish with parsley sprigs. Serve immediately.

Serves 4. Per serving: 148 Calories; 9g Fat, 13g Protein, 3g Carbohydrate; 1g dietary fiber.

QUICK COFFEE CUP SCRAMBLE

Be certain to coat the coffee mug with cooking spray to ensure easy clean up. Never be limited in your mug creations. The method and base ingredients are a perfect host to countless ingredients and flavors.

Ingredients:
Cooking Spray
2 eggs
2 Tablespoons milk
2 Tablespoons Cheddar cheese, shredded
Pepper, to taste
Finishing salt, to taste

Coat a 12-ounce microwave-safe coffee mug with cooking spray. Add eggs and milk; beat with a fork until blended. Microwave on High 45 seconds; remove and stir. Microwave until eggs are almost set, 30 to 45 seconds longer. Top with cheese; season with pepper and finishing salt. Cool slightly before eating warm.

Serves 1. Per serving: 224 Calories; 16g Fat; 17g Protein; 2g Carbohydrate.

MUGGY EGGS BREAKFAST BAR

I'm using the term "breakfast bar" loosely to describe the advance preparation of ingredients to make the creation of a morning egg mug a breeze. Consider gathering any of the ingredients listed –or anything you enjoy – to keep on hand in the refrigerator. Organize breakfast bar ingredients in easy-to-access containers or resealable plastic bags and store in one location for easy access. With a few select items and a dozen eggs you can have a warm protein first meal to start the day, even on the most hectic mornings. Simply use a few supplies and the basic method for cooking microwave mug eggs and build your original breakfast creation one scrumptious mug at a time. For example, chop left-over fried chicken, add to eggs, top with ready-to-eat country gravy and enjoy a breakfast so yummy you'll be happy all day long!

Try these great Variations:

Animal protein: cooked ground meat; cooked steak or pork chops, sliced; cooked shredded poultry; chopped Canadian bacon; cooked sausage, crumbled and drained; bacon, cooked drained of fat and crumbled; canned fish; cooked fish fillets, flaked; deli meat, sliced and chopped; seafood including shrimp, scallops, lobster, etc., cooked and chopped.

Dairy: eggs, cottage cheese; sour cream; assorted varieties shredded cheese; milk; butter; pasteurized egg product (Egg Beaters®).

Vegetables: Any cooked vegetables including asparagus; bell peppers; broccoli; carrots; cooked greens (chard, spinach, kale); sautéed celery or fennel; legumes including canned beans and canned refried beans; mushrooms; onions or leeks; snow peas; green and yellow snap beans; tomatoes both raw and cooked (canned); summer squash (zucchini, crookneck; cooked and mashed winter squash (acorn, banana, butternut, pumpkin, and spaghetti squash).

Condiments: salsa, green chili sauce, spaghetti, marinara, and alfredo sauce, tapenade, bruschetta-style tomato sauce, pesto, hummus, mayonnaise, mustard, ketchup, gravy (ready-to-serve), assorted vinaigrettes and salad dressings.

Helpful Hints and Tips: Double-check the mug or bowl intended for cooking your eggs to ensure it is safe for microwave cooking. Use hot pads to handle mugs and bowls which become quite hot during cooking.

Always use cooking spray to liberally coat the inside of the mug or bowl before microwave cooking eggs. Try olive oil or butter flavored sprays. Cooking spray is the best ingredient to use to prevent stuck-on eggs that make clean-up nearly impossible.

If you enjoy sautéed vegetables in your eggs cook a batch on the weekend; store refrigerated in a tightly covered container; add by the spoonful to your mug egg concoction during the week. (I like a mixture of chopped onion, celery, bell pepper, and mushrooms.) Leftover vegetables can also serve this purpose.

Fresh fruit or berries are a sweet and flavorful side dish compliment to the Basic Microwave Coffee Cup Scramble. Including a few bites of melon, strawberries, grapes and other fresh fruits and berries is a smart strategy for preempting sugar cravings later in the morning.

For a boost of energy in the afternoon make a coffee mug scramble. The protein will satisfy hunger cravings and provide an energy boost without the negative "carb-coma" effect of a non-nutritional simple carbohydrate snack.

ITALIAN VEGETABLE EGG CUSTARD

Custard doesn't have to be sweet to be delicious. This savory brunch custard makes great use of fresh summer vegetables. After you have tried it with squash and tomatoes, experiment with other fresh vegetables like peppers, mushrooms, and even diced or shredded winter squash. Explore your creative Receptiveness! See page 74.

Ingredients:
Cooking spray
4 eggs
1/2 cup all-purpose flour

2 cups summer squash, shredded
1 cup zucchini, shredded
1/2 cup black olives, sliced, divided
2 Tablespoons Parmesan cheese, grated
1 teaspoon Italian seasoning
½-teaspoon garlic salt
1 medium tomato, thinly sliced
1 bunch green onions, sliced 1/2-inch thick
½-cup mozzarella cheese, shredded

Preheat the oven to 450°F and place the rack in the middle of the oven. Spray an 8-inch square baking pan with cooking spray. In a medium bowl beat the eggs and flour until smooth. Stir in summer squash, zucchini and 1/4 cup olives; mix well. Spread in prepared baking pan. Place in center of oven and bake until custard is set, about 10 minutes. (see note). Remove to a warm trivet.

Mix the Parmesan cheese, Italian seasoning and garlic salt together and sprinkle evenly over the baked custard. Top evenly with tomato slices, remaining olives, sliced green onion and mozzarella cheese. Divide into four equal portions and serve warm.

Note: To determine that the custard is done insert a wooden skewer or toothpick into the center about two-thirds down. If it comes out clean the custard is done. If the custard is almost done turn the oven off and leave the oven door slightly ajar so the custard will finish cooking

Serves 4. Per serving: 232 Calories; 12g Fat; 13g Protein; 19g Carbohydrate; 3g Dietary Fiber.

MUSHROOM-TOPPED EGG CUPS

These are easy to make appetizers for a party, but I enjoy them for breakfast. You can vary the toppings with fresh seasonal produce. Serve with berries or melon.

Ingredients:
Cooking spray
12 each wonton skins (see note)

2 eggs
1 cup half and half
¼-teaspoon salt
Dash pepper
1/2 cup button mushrooms, sliced
1/2 cup ham, diced
1/2 cup Cheddar cheese, shredded
1/2 cup mozzarella cheese, shredded
2 ounces pimiento, sliced
2 Tablespoons parsley, chopped

Preheat the oven to 375°F and place the rack in the center of the oven. Spray a 12-cup muffin pan with cooking spray. Press one wonton skin into each cup, forming to cup. Set aside.

In a bowl whisk together the eggs, half-and-half, salt, and pepper. Divide evenly among muffin cups. Top each cup with mushrooms, ham, Cheddar cheese, and mozzarella cheese. Top evenly with pimiento and parsley. Bake for 15 minutes or until a knife inserted near the centers comes out clean. Serve warm.

Serves 6: two eggcups per serving. Per serving: 170 Calories; 13g Fat; 10g Protein; 3g Carbohydrate; trace Dietary Fiber.

*Note: Wonton skins are paper-thin squares of dough made from flour, water, eggs, and salt. They are used to make wontons, egg rolls and other crispy Chinese dishes. They are found in the produce section of most supermarkets. When working with wonton skins keep them covered with moist paper toweling to prevent drying.

CHEESY SCRAMBLED EGGS

This creamy egg dish reheats well. Make it on the weekend and divide into individual serving dishes for a quick breakfast during the workweek. Gently reheat in the microwave oven. Use reduced fat cream cheese if desired.

Ingredients:
12 large eggs
¼-teaspoon pepper
6 Tablespoons butter or margarine
6 ounces tub-style cream cheese with chives and onions, diced

In a large bowl, beat eggs and pepper until just blended. In a large 12-inch skillet over medium-high heat, melt butter or margarine. Add egg mixture. As egg mixture begins to set, stir slightly with a rubber spatula so the uncooked egg flows to bottom. When eggs are partially cooked add diced cream cheese. Continue cooking until egg mixture is set but still moist, stirring occasionally.

Serves 8. Per serving: 258 Calories; 22g Fat; 11g Protein; 2g Carbohydrate; trace Dietary Fiber.

SCANDINAVIAN COUNTRY-STYLE SCRAMBLED EGGS

Cardamom is a member of the ginger family and is native to India. The spicy-sweet flavor is typical in both East Indian and Scandinavian cuisines. Cardamom can be purchased in pod form or ground. The pods, about the size of a cranberry, hold the seeds that become the spice. To use the seeds from the pod simply crush with a mortar and pestle or the back of knife to release the seeds. You can add both the seeds and papery shell to your dish: the shell will dissolve. If you are not familiar with the strong spicy-sweet flavor of cardamom use it prudently: a little goes a long way.

Ingredients:
6 eggs
¼-teaspoon cardamom, ground
Cooking spray
2 teaspoons butter
1 Tablespoon flour
12 ounces evaporated milk*, canned, room temperature
Salt and pepper, to taste.

In a medium bowl whisk the eggs together until broken and blended, but not frothy. Whisk in the cardamom and set aside. Spray a medium 10-inch skillet with cooking spray and place over medium heat. Add the butter and melt; stir in the flour and whisk until blended. Slowly, while whisking, pour in the evaporated milk and continue to whisk the sauce until thickened and coats the back of a spoon. Whisk the eggs into the sauce and cook gently until eggs are set, about 4 to 6 minutes. Season with salt and pepper, to taste. Serve warm. Optional: use freshly ground nutmeg in place of the cardamom.

Serves 4. Per serving: 250 Calories; 16g Fat; 15g Protein; 11g Carbohydrate; trace Dietary Fiber.

*I use evaporated milk in this recipe. It has been heated to remove 60 percent of the water contained in pasteurized milk making it richer and creamier. It contains more protein and calcium per serving than fresh milk.

CLASSIC OMELETS

A traditional French omelet is a mixture of eggs, seasonings and sometimes water or milk, cooked in butter until firm and filled or topped with various fillings such as cheese, ham, mushrooms, onions, peppers, sausage and herbs. There are no definitive rules with omelets, so the cook has the pleasure of filling this light airy egg mixture with the things they enjoy. Omelet stations are popular at brunch buffets and a good choice for the weight loss surgery patient who can request a custom prepared omelet.

Omelet making can feel intimidating if you have watched a television or restaurant chef wiggle and flip the pan to perfection. But with a little practice home cooks can master the technique; I'm still working on it. Use a good quality non-stick pan and coat it with butter, oil or cooking spray. Make sure the oil is hot before proceeding to add the eggs and then keep things moving. Serve fresh tomato and avocado slices on the side for a delicious well-rounded omelet brunch.

SPINACH, HAM & CHEESE OMELET

Ingredients:
2 eggs
2 Tablespoons water
Cooking spray
1 teaspoon butter
Salt and pepper, to taste
1/4 cup mozzarella cheese, shredded

1/4 cup spinach leaves, chopped
1/4 cup ham slices, extra lean, chopped

Beat eggs and water in a small bowl until blended. Heat butter in a small 8-inch nonstick omelet pan or skillet over medium high heat until hot. Tilt pan to coat bottom. Pour in egg mixture. Mixture should set immediately at the edges.

Gently push cooked portions from edges toward the center with inverted turner so that uncooked eggs can reach the hot pan surface. Continue cooking, tilting pan and gently moving cooked portions as needed.

When top surface of eggs is thickened and no visible liquid egg remains, season with salt and pepper. Place cheese on one side of omelet; top with spinach and ham. Fold omelet in half with turner. With a quick flip of the wrist, turn pan and invert or slide omelet onto plate. Serve immediately.

Serves 2. Per serving: 176 Calories; 12g Fat; 15g Protein; 1g Carbohydrate; trace Dietary Fiber.

OLIVE & RED PEPPER OMELET

For more servings multiply the ingredients by the number of servings you require. Making each omelet individually produces the best results. Whisk all of the eggs and water together and then use 1/2 cup of egg mixture for each omelet.

Ingredients:
Cooking spray
2 Tablespoons roasted red peppers, chopped
1 Tablespoon onion flakes
Pinch garlic salt
2 eggs
2 Tablespoons water
1 Tablespoon parsley sprigs, chopped
2 Tablespoons sharp Cheddar cheese, shredded
1 Tablespoon black olives, sliced

In a medium 7 to 10-inch skillet heat the cooking spray over medium heat. Add the roasted red pepper, the onion flakes, and garlic salt. Meanwhile whisk together the eggs and water until blended.

Pour into skillet with peppers. The eggs should set immediately at the edges. Gently push cooked portions from edges toward the center with inverted turner so that uncooked eggs can reach the hot pan surface. Continue cooking, tilting pan and gently moving cooked portions as needed. When the top surface of eggs is thickened and no visible liquid egg remains, sprinkle with cheese and olives. Fold omelet in half with turner. With a quick flip of the wrist, turn pan and invert or slide omelet onto plate. Serve immediately.

Serves 1. Per serving: 89 Calories; 16g Fat; 17g Protein; 7g Carbohydrate; 1g Dietary Fiber.

TOFU & VEGGIE BREAKFAST SCRAMBLE

Tofu is a versatile food that is remarkably nutritious. It is a complete protein and rich in minerals. A soy product, tofu is believed to contain cancer-fighting substances. In North America we shy away from tofu because it is strange, but once we get become familiar with tofu, we find it takes on a variety of flavors and can be creatively included in our high protein diet.

Ingredients:
2 Tablespoons olive oil
1 medium onion, chopped
1 medium red bell pepper, chopped
12 button mushrooms, sliced
2 cloves garlic, minced
12 ounces tofu*, firm, cubed 1-inch squares
1 Tablespoon soy sauce, low sodium
1 Tablespoon all-purpose seasoning blend
1 bunch spinach, chopped
1 cup salsa, optional, room temperature

Heat the olive oil in a large 12-inch skillet over medium heat until hot. Add the onion, red bell pepper, button mushrooms and garlic. Cook and stir until vegetables are translucent and tender. Add tofu, soy sauce, all-purpose seasoning blend and continue to cook and stir gently for about 3 minutes. Add spinach greens and continue to cook and stir until spinach is wilted. Serve warm, topped with salsa if desired.

Serves 4. Per serving: 218 Calories; 11g Fat; 13g Protein; 22g Carbohydrate; 5g Dietary Fiber.

*Tofu, sometimes called "the cheese of Asia", is a good source of vegetable protein derived from soy. Recent research indicates that soy protein may help lower total cholesterol levels and reduce the tendency of platelets to form blood clots. The nature of tofu to take on other flavors makes it easy to include in the diet without grave palate panic. Slowly adding tofu is a good idea. In this recipe you could use 6-ounces tofu and 3 eggs, beaten, and prepare as directed before going for all-out tofu. The change will hardly be noticeable, except, perhaps, to the health of your heart.

POULTRY

As lifelong dieters we are familiar with the benefits of poultry: lean nutrient-dense protein, inexpensive, readily available, quick and easy to prepare. The challenge we face is keeping it interesting. We also must prepare it in a manner to keep it moist enough to be tolerated by our sensitive gastric pouch while keeping it palatable and satiating to our mouth. And we probably need to feed others the same thing we are eating. That's a tall order for the humble bird.

On average 3 ounces of cooked chicken (white and dark meat without the skin) provides 162 Calories; 25g Protein; 6g Fat (2g saturated); 76mg Cholesterol and 73mg Sodium. Chicken is a good source of nutrients including niacin, vitamin B6, and zinc.

SKILLET CHICKEN PARMESAN

This is a favorite go-to recipe around our house. In the cool days of autumn, I like to serve it with baked spaghetti squash. A fresh green salad also goes nicely with this nutrient rich meal.

Ingredients:
olive oil flavored cooking spray
4 (4-ounce) chicken breasts, no skin, no bone, Ready-to-Cook
1 (26-ounce jar) marinara sauce
4 ounces mozzarella cheese, part skim milk, shredded
1/4 cup Parmesan cheese

Coat a 10-inch skillet with olive oil spray and heat over medium-high heat. Add the chicken breasts and cook 6 minutes. Turn and continue cooking.

Pour marinara sauce over chicken, reduce heat and simmer, uncovered, for 10 minutes. Divide the mozzarella cheese and Parmesan cheese evenly over the chicken pieces. Remove skillet from heat, cover and let stand 5 minutes or until the cheese is melted. Serve warm.

Serves 4. Per serving: 341 Calories, 13g Fat; 16g Carbohydrate. Dark meat chicken is an excellent source of niacin.

APPLE GLAZED TURKEY TENDERLOIN

Turkey contains tryptophan, the amino acid blamed for Thanksgiving Day naps. But did you know that tryptophan helps us synthesize the vitamin niacin to produce serotonin, a neurotransmitter important in sleep regulation, appetite control and sensory perception. Serve this dish with cooked frozen peas and pearl onions tossed with melted apple jelly and a pinch of sage.

Ingredients:
Cooking spray
1 (1 pound) turkey breast tenderloin*
1 Tablespoon lemon juice
1 Tablespoon olive oil
2 cloves garlic, minced
½-teaspoon coarse salt
½-teaspoon dried sage, crushed
2 Tablespoons apple jelly, melted

Preheat broiler. Line broiler tray with heavy-duty aluminum foil and place rack on top. Spray with cooking spray. Split turkey breast tenderloin in half horizontally, open, and place on prepared broiler pan. In a small bowl combine lemon juice, olive oil, garlic, coarse salt, and sage. Brush lemon mixture on both sides of each turkey piece.

Broil turkey 4 to 5 inches from the heat for 5 minutes. Turn turkey; broil for 2 minutes more. Brush turkey with apple jelly. Broil for 2 to 3-minutes more or until turkey is tender and no longer pink. Remove the tenderloin to a warm platter and let rest 5 minutes. Slice on the diagonal and serve with additional apple jelly.

Serves 4. Per serving: 170 Calories; 4g Fat; 24g Protein; 7g Carbohydrate; trace Dietary Fiber.

*Several cuts of turkey are available in the fresh poultry section of the supermarket. Look for tenderloin and breast cutlets that have not been injected with additives or phosphates. As always watch expiration dates and observe safe food handling practices. See the Appendix for a safe food-handling guide.

BASIL CHICKEN CURRY WITH LIME

This is curry in a hurry without leaving home and with knowing exactly what you are eating. Great for the entire family! Thai cooking is something I have introduced to our DAY 6 DIET only after weight loss surgery. The dishes tend to be spicy and sweet at the same time, which is a proven combination to bring satiation to the palate. You can take the level of spice heat up or down in this recipe by adjusting the amount of curry paste you use. Also look for curry paste labeled mild, hot or extra hot and buy according to your personal preference. By combining equal parts coconut milk and low-fat evaporated milk we can lower the fat and still enjoy the classic flavor of coconut in this curry.

Ingredients:
2 teaspoons sesame oil
1 Tablespoon curry paste
2 cloves garlic, minced
1 medium onion, cut into wedges
1 1/2 pounds boneless chicken, cut into strips
1 medium red bell pepper, cut into strips
4 ounces button mushrooms, sliced
3/4 cup coconut milk
3/4 cup low-fat evaporated milk
1 medium lime, juiced
1 cup basil leaves, loosely packed
Pepper, to taste

In a large 12-inch skillet or wok heat the sesame oil over medium-high heat until hot. Add curry paste and stir for 1 minute to soften. Add garlic and onion and cook and stir quickly for 2-3 minutes or until the onion is translucent. Push the onion and garlic to the sides of the skillet and add chicken. Lightly brown chicken on all sides.

Add red bell pepper, mushrooms, coconut milk, evaporated milk, lime juice, basil and pepper and stir all ingredients together well. Continue cooking until chicken is cooked through, about 5 minutes. The sauce should be slightly reduced. Serve warm.

Serves 4. Per serving: 410 Calories; 18g Fat 46g Protein; 17g Carbohydrate; 3g Dietary Fiber.

CHICKEN WITH APPLES & BLUE CHEESE

This is a good weeknight meal to enjoy when the apples are at their best in the fall. The blue cheese is a savory compliment to the sweet-tart Granny Smith apples. Look for firm apples with a shiny skin and free of blemishes or bruises. Serve additional apple slices to complete the meal.

Chicken thighs contain a higher concentration of minerals, including zinc and iron, than the more popular chicken breasts. The meat is richly flavored and tender with fewer tendencies to dry out. Most major supermarkets carry bulk bags of frozen ready-to-eat boneless skinless chicken thighs. A 3-ounce cooked serving of dark meat chicken contains 166 calories and 21 grams of protein.

Ingredients:
Cooking spray
1 1/4 pounds boneless, skinless chicken thighs
2 teaspoons poultry seasoning
1/2 medium onion, chopped
1 medium Granny Smith apple, peeled, cored, sliced
1/2 cup chicken broth
2 Tablespoons blue cheese, crumbled
Salt and pepper, to taste

Coat a deep large 12-inch skillet with cooking spray and heat over medium-high heat. Season the chicken with the poultry seasoning and add to hot pan. Reduce heat to medium and cook 4 to 6 minutes per side or until no longer pink in the center. Transfer to a platter and tent with foil to keep warm. Return skillet to medium high heat.

Add the onions and apples to the skillet and cook and stir for 2 minutes. Add the broth and continue cooking until reduced and the apples are tender. Add any accumulated juices from the chicken platter and cook 1 minute longer. Divide the chicken evenly onto 4 plates. Top equally with the apples, onions and sauce, and garnish each serving with 1/2 tablespoon blue cheese crumbles. Serve warm.

Serves 4. Per serving: 200 Calories; 4g Fat; 35g Protein; 5g Carbohydrate; 1g Dietary Fiber.

COCONUT CHICKEN NUGGETS

Packaged coconut is available in cans or plastic bags, sweetened or unsweetened, shredded or flaked, and dried, moist or frozen. It can sometimes also be found toasted. Unopened canned coconut can be stored at room temperature up to 18 months; coconut in plastic bags up to six months. Refrigerate both after opening. Coconut is high in saturated fat and is a good source of potassium. Serve these tasty chicken nuggets with tossed greens topped with mango, pineapple, coconut flakes and macadamia nuts and drizzled with light vinaigrette.

Ingredients:
Cooking spray
1 1/2 pounds boneless, skinless chicken, white or dark meat
1 cup unsweetened coconut flakes
3/4 cup panko*
1/4 cup butter or margarine, melted
Salt and pepper, to taste

Preheat oven to 375°F and place the rack in the center of the oven. Line a rimmed baking sheet with heavy-duty foil and spray liberally with cooking spray.

Cut boneless chicken into bite size pieces, about 1 1/2-inch cubed. In a shallow dish stir together coconut and panko. Toss chicken cubes in the melted butter, season with salt and pepper to taste and roll in coconut-panko mixture. Place chicken pieces on prepared baking sheet making sure they do not touch. Bake for 15-20 minutes until chicken is tender and no longer pink. Do not turn chicken pieces while baking. Serve warm.

Serves 6. Per serving: 313 Calories; 18g Fat; 28g Protein; 9g Carbohydrate; 2g Dietary Fiber.

*Panko are Japanese breadcrumbs that are coarser than traditional American breadcrumbs. They are a good choice for us because a light coating works to satisfy that crunch-craving we get from time-to-time. Even when baked in the oven they produce a delightful crispy crunch without sacrificing nutrition.

ITALIAN-STYLE TURKEY MEATLOAF WITH SPAGHETTI SQUASH

Ingredients:
Cooking spray
1 1/4 pounds ground turkey
1 1/4 pounds turkey sausage
1/2 cup breadcrumbs
1 egg
1 cup marinara sauce, divided
1 clove garlic, minced
1 teaspoon Italian seasoning blend

Preheat oven to 350°F. Line a rimmed baking sheet with foil and spray liberally with cooking spray. In a large bowl, combine ground turkey, turkey sausage, breadcrumbs, egg, 1/2 cup marinara sauce, garlic and Italian seasoning blend. Mix well.

On the prepared baking sheet shape the mixture into a rectangular loaf. Spread top with remaining marinara sauce. Bake for 1 hour or until no longer pink in the center and internal temperature of loaf reaches 165°F. Let stand at room temperature 5 minutes before slicing.

Serves 6. Per serving: 214 Calories; 10g Fat; 19g Protein; 10g Carbohydrate; 1g Dietary Fiber.

BAKED SPAGHETTI SQUASH

1 1/2 pounds spaghetti squash
2 Tablespoons butter
1 1/2 cups marinara sauce
3 Tablespoons Parmesan cheese, grated

Keeping squash whole, pierce skin with a carving fork in several places. Wrap in heavy-duty aluminum foil. Place in the heated 350°F oven. Prepare the Turkey Meatloaf and bake as directed alongside the squash. While meatloaf rests, remove the squash from the oven and carefully remove the foil avoiding steam burns: cool. When cool enough to handle cut in half lengthwise and remove seeds and strings from hollow center. Then, with a fork, pull the "spaghetti" from the shell of the squash. Place on a platter and dab with pats of butter. Heat the Marinara sauce for 2 to 3 minutes in microwave oven set to medium. Stir and spoon over spaghetti squash. Sprinkle with Parmesan cheese.

Serves 6. Per serving: 116 Calories; 7g Fat; 3g Protein; 13g Carbohydrate; 1g Dietary Fiber.

PEANUT CRUSTED BAKED CHICKEN WITH PEANUT SAUCE

This is a new take on the perennial favorite chicken nuggets. I have never had a child turn away from this easy, tasty meal. But then again, I've never seen an adult turn away either. Make this meal complete with a fresh green salad topped with mandarin oranges, a few honey-roasted peanuts and a drizzle of the peanut sauce.

Ingredients:
Cooking spray
4 ounces honey-roasted peanuts
1 egg
1/2 cup milk, 2% low-fat
1 1/2 pounds boneless chicken, cut into strips
1 package A Taste of Thai Peanut Sauce Mix, prepared as directed

Preheat the oven to 350°F and place the rack in the center of the oven. Spray a foil lined baking sheet liberally with cooking spray.

In the bowl of a food processor grind the honey-roasted peanuts until course. Place in a shallow pie plate. In another shallow pie plate whisk together the egg and milk. Dip the chicken strips in the milk and then dredge in the honey-roasted peanuts. Place on the prepared baking sheet one inch apart. Bake the chicken strips for 18 to 20 minutes and test for doneness.

While the chicken strips bake prepare the Thai Peanut Sauce Mix according to package directions. Serve sauce in a dipping bowl on the side.

Serves 4. Per serving: 390 Calories; 18g Fat; 48g Protein; 10g Carbohydrate; 2g Dietary Fiber.

Peanuts are a healthy source of monounsaturated fats, which are believed to promote heart health. Peanuts are a legume, not a nut. Studies indicate that when included in a healthy diet the risk of cardiovascular disease is reduced by an estimated 21 percent compared to the average American diet.

THAI-CURRIED GAME HENS

Jim calls Cornish game hens "little chickens". I just call them delicious. Game hens are inexpensive and usually only available frozen. They average 12 ounces each and are rich in B vitamins and protein. Normally I cook them with the skin on to retain moisture, but I eat only the meat. A University of Minnesota study found that no significant fat is transferred from the skin to the meat when poultry is cooked. So when roasting, broiling, or grilling poultry it's okay to leave the skin on during cooking as long as the skin is removed before eating.

Ingredients:
3 Tablespoons canola oil, divided
2 teaspoons Thai Red curry paste
1 Tablespoon tomato paste
1 cup coconut milk, unsweetened
1 cup low-sodium chicken broth
1 can (15-ounces) straw mushrooms, drained
2 Tablespoons fish sauce
1 Tablespoon brown sugar, packed

6 medium cherry tomatoes, quartered

2 (11-ounce) game hens, thawed, giblets removed

Heat 1 tablespoon olive oil in a large 12-inch skillet over medium heat. Add curry paste and tomato paste and stir until fragrant, about 3 minutes. Add coconut milk, broth, mushrooms, fish sauce, and brown sugar. Bring to a simmer. Remove from heat. Add cherry tomatoes. Season sauce with salt and pepper to taste.

Preheat oven to 350°F. Heat remaining 2 tablespoons oil in large nonstick skillet. Add game hens and cook until browned, about 4 minutes per side. Transfer hens to 13x9x2-inch glass or ceramic baking dish. Pour sauce over. Bake uncovered until hens are cooked through, about 35 minutes. Transfer hens to shallow serving bowl; tent with foil. Skim fat from sauce. Pour sauce into large skillet; boil 5 minutes. Pour sauce over hens. Serve warm.

Serves 4. Per Serving: 448 Calories; 32g Fat; 31g Protein; 14g Carbohydrate; 2g Dietary Fiber.

Thyme & Garlic Chicken Breasts and Asparagus Parmesan

This easy slow cooker recipe calls for bone-in chicken breasts. If you prefer use one whole fryer chicken cut into pieces.

Ingredients:

6 chicken breast halves, without skin, frozen*

1 clove garlic, minced

1 1/2 teaspoons dried thyme, crushed

1/4 cup orange juice

1 Tablespoon balsamic vinegar

Place chicken in a 3 1/2- or 4-quart slow cooker. Season with garlic and thyme. Pour orange juice and balsamic vinegar over chicken. Cover and cook on low heat setting for 5 to 6 hours or on high heat setting for 2 1/2 to 3 hours. Transfer chicken to a serving platter, reserving juices. Cover chicken; keep warm.

For sauce, skim off fat from cooking juices. Strain juices into a small saucepan. Bring to boiling; reduce heat. Boil gently, uncovered, about 10 minutes or until reduced to about 1 cup. Serve sauce with chicken.

Serves 6. Per serving: 207 Calories; 2g Fat; 42g Protein; 2g Carbohydrate; trace Dietary Fiber.

*Note: I found that using frozen poultry in the slow cooker results in a perfectly tender cooked piece of meat. Fresh or thawed poultry tends to get rubbery after all-day cooking in the slow cooker.

ROASTED ASPARAGUS PARMESAN

Some gastric surgery patients report discomfort from eating asparagus. Peeling the outer scales with a vegetable peeler can reduce the amount of stringy fiber that is the cause of gastric upset.

Ingredients:

2 pounds asparagus

2 Tablespoons olive oil spray

1 teaspoon Provence seasoning blend

1/2 cup Parmesan cheese, grated

Preheat oven to 400°F and place rack in center. Wash asparagus spears and pat dry. Snap off and discard wood bases from asparagus. Place asparagus in a 15x10x1-inch baking pan. Coat with olive oil spray and season with Provence seasoning blend. Toss gently to coat.

Roast in oven for about 15 minutes or until asparagus is crisp-tender. While asparagus roasts make sauce for chicken. Transfer to a serving platter; sprinkle with Parmesan cheese. Serve warm with Garlic Thyme Chicken Breasts.

Serves 6. Per serving: 91 Calories; 7g Fat; 5g Protein; 4g Carbohydrate; 2g Dietary Fiber.

There's no greater satisfaction than cooking a perfectly roasted chicken. -- Art Smith

SUNDAY SUPPER ROAST CHICKEN AND VEGETABLES

This is one of those throw together recipes that is robust with flavor and wholesome goodness. Like so many others we open our doors on Sunday nights and all who enter are welcome to sit at our table. This is the perfect meal for casual gatherings. It lends itself well to all manner of personalization. Find the things you like, the ingredients that are fresh and seasonal. Let the oven do the work for you and let food bring together the people you care about. I take some help from the store with prepared mashed potatoes, gravy and rolls. It is more important to me to spend time with family and friends on Sunday afternoon than it is to spend time in the kitchen. I hope you'll enjoy this Sunday Supper.

Ingredients:
2 large roasting chickens
1-pound carrots, washed, peeled, chunked
8 celery ribs, washed, chunked
2 large yellow onions, quartered
1-pound potatoes, quartered
1-pound button mushrooms, wiped clean
Olive oil
Salt and pepper, to taste
2 packages prepared mashed potatoes
2 jars chicken gravy
1 dozen bakery rolls

Line a large roasting pan with heavy-duty foil for easy clean up. Preheat the oven to 350-375°F. Place the vegetables in the bottom of the roasting pan and toss with a small amount of olive oil, not too much because the chicken will release oil. Season lightly with salt and pepper and toss again.

Prepare the chicken according to package directions (some will contain giblet or gravy mixes, some will not) and place directly atop the vegetable mixture. Place in heated oven uncovered. Cook for 90 minutes to 2 hours or until internal temperature at thigh measures 170°F or pop-up thermometer indicates chicken is done. Remove from oven and place chickens on platter to rest, tenting loosely with foil. The vegetables should be nicely caramelized, scoop them to a serving bowl. Cover to keep warm.

Heat the prepared mashed potatoes following package directions, transfer to a pretty serving bowl. In a small saucepot heat prepared chicken gravy to a gentle simmer. Transfer to a gravy boat or serving bowl. Place bakery rolls in a towel-lined breadbasket. Carve the chickens and arrange on platter. Invite your guests to join you for a beautiful Sunday supper. Serve fresh seasonal fruit or berries for dessert. Wine is optional. Cheers!

FISH & SHELLFISH

Fish and shellfish are excellent sources of lean protein, and according to the American Heart Association, they are good for the old ticker too. According to the AHA we should include two servings of fish a week in our diet. The AHA advises eating fish relatively high in omega-3 fatty acids including salmon, trout and herring. We should grill, bake or poach fish and limit commercially fried fish. In addition, fish should be prepared without added salt, saturated and trans-fat.

Mild fish, such as snapper, striped bass, and rainbow trout are rich in omega-3 fatty acids in addition to B12, magnesium, vitamin B6, niacin, potassium and vitamin E. On average they contain around 140 calories per serving and nearly 30g Protein per serving.

Shellfish, such as shrimp, are low-fat yet nutrient rich containing vitamin B12, iron, niacin, zinc and copper. They contain 112 calories per 4 ounce serving and 24 grams of protein.

Quality flash-frozen fish is available in the freezer section, individually wrapped in pre-measured 4-ounce servings with eight to ten servings per package. This is convenient for thawing only the portions needed for a single meal.

When buying fresh fish look for flesh that is moist and slightly translucent; the flesh should feel resilient and there should be no fishy odor. Fresh fish should be displayed on ice. Saltwater fish, such as tuna, may have a pleasant saltwater smell.

After visiting Alaska our Neighbors gave us some halibut they captured along with this recipe. I like this chowder recipe because it is not as heavy as many New England chowders and it does not include potatoes, which are too starchy for me. The addition of sharp Cheddar cheese makes this recipe especially rich. A one-cup serving is plenty to keep me full and happy for hours.

Have all your ingredients prepared before starting the cooking process: the recipe comes together quite quickly. You may wish to serve crusty bread for the starch eaters in your family.

Ingredients:
2 pounds Alaska halibut, thawed if frozen
1/2 medium onion, finely chopped
1 green bell pepper, finely chopped
4 ribs celery, finely chopped
4 whole carrots, peeled and finely chopped
6 Tablespoons butter or margarine, room temperature, divided
3 cups chicken broth
1-teaspoon salt
½-teaspoon white pepper
2 cups dairy milk
3 Tablespoons all-purpose flour
12 ounces (2½-cups) sharp Cheddar cheese, shredded
1 Tablespoon minced parsley

Remove skin and bones from halibut; cut into bite-sized pieces. Cook and stir vegetables in 3 tablespoons butter until vegetables are tender. Add halibut, chicken broth, salt and pepper. Simmer covered, 5 minutes. Add milk and heat gently. Combine remaining 3 tablespoons butter with flour and add to chowder. Cook and stir until slightly thickened. Add cheese; cook and stir over low heat until cheese melts. Garnish with parsley.

Serves 6-8. Per Serving: 418 Calories; 26g Fat; 37g Protein; 9g Carbohydrate; 1g Dietary Fiber.

BROILED SALMON STEAKS WITH LEMON & ORANGE

Fresh or frozen salmon may be used in this recipe. Adjust quantities to provide a 4-ounce serving for each person. Salmon is rich in omega-3 fatty acids, which are believed to lower triglycerides and may also fight cancer and reduce inflammation. Serve with Spinach Salad & Orange Vinaigrette.

Ingredients:
Cooking spray
2 (4-ounce) salmon fillets, fresh or frozen
1 teaspoon lemon peel, finely grated
1 tablespoon lemon juice
1 clove garlic, minced
1/4-teaspoon black pepper
1 Tablespoon green onion, sliced
1 medium orange, peeled and sliced

Thaw fish, if frozen. Preheat broiler. Line broiler pan with heavy-duty aluminum foil and place rack on top. Spray liberally with cooking spray. In a small bowl stir together lemon peel, lemon juice, garlic, and pepper.

Rinse fish; pat dry with paper towels. Place fish on the prepared broiler rack. Brush with half of the lemon juice mixture. Broil about 4 inches from the heat for 5 minutes. Turn fish; brush with the remaining lemon juice mixture. Broil for 3 to 7 minutes more or until fish flakes easily when tested with a fork. Place warm salmon on plates and garnish with green onion and serve with orange slices. Serve with Spinach Salad.

Serves 2. Per serving: 168 Calories; 23g Protein; 9g Carbohydrate; 2g Dietary Fiber.

SPINACH SALAD WITH ORANGE VINAIGRETTE

In a small bowl whisk together 1 tablespoon orange juice, 1 tablespoon walnut oil, 1 tablespoon white-wine vinegar, 1/4 teaspoon orange zest, salt and freshly ground black pepper to taste. Toss with 2 cups fresh baby spinach, 1 navel orange, peeled and cut into bite-size pieces, 1/4 cup dried cranberries, and 1 Tablespoon chopped toasted walnuts.

Fresh crabmeat is the first choice for this recipe. However, pasteurized crabmeat is an acceptable and convenient alternative. The ready to use crabmeat is sold in sealed container in refrigerator section at the market. Look for tubs of fresh, never frozen, crabmeat. Check the expiration date: once opened crabmeat has a shelf life of 2-3 days under refrigeration. Crab is an excellent source of copper and zinc. Serve with salad greens a fresh-diced avocado.

Although the ingredient list is long, this recipe comes together quite easily with the help of a food processor. It is an excellent weekend treat for brunch or a late afternoon lunch. Serve it with a crisp green salad and melon for dessert.

Sauce:

1/2 medium California avocado
1 Tablespoon Miracle Whip® light
1 Tablespoon lime juice
¼-teaspoon salt
¼-teaspoon sugar
1 medium mild chile (or jalapeno)
1/4 cup milk, 1% low-fat

Crab Cakes:

16-ounces crabmeat, picked over and coarsely shredded
3 Tablespoons Miracle Whip® light
1/4 cup chives, minced
1 Tablespoon lemon juice
1 teaspoon Dijon-style mustard
¼-teaspoon black pepper
1/2 cup panko (Japanese Breadcrumbs), divided
1 Tablespoon butter, unsalted
2 cloves garlic, smashed
½-teaspoon Provence seasoning blend
¼-teaspoon salt

Preheat oven to 400°F and position rack in middle. For Sauce: Pulse avocado with Miracle Whip® light, lime juice, salt, sugar, and one fourth of chile in a food processor until blended. Add milk and puree until smooth. Add more chiles, to taste. Transfer sauce to a bowl and chill, covered. Stir together crabmeat, Miracle Whip® light, chives, lemon juice, mustard, pepper, and 1 tablespoon panko in a large bowl until blended well, then chill, covered.

Melt butter in a small 8-inch skillet over medium heat. Add garlic and cook until fragrant, about 2 minutes. Add Provence seasoning blend, salt and remaining 7 tablespoons panko and cook, stirring, until crumbs are golden brown, about 6 minutes. Transfer crumbs to a plate and cool. Discard garlic.

Divide crabmeat mixture into four mounds and form into patties. Carefully turn patty into crumb mixture to coat top and bottom. Transfer to a baking sheet and repeat with remaining 3 mounds, then sprinkle remaining crumbs on top of crab cakes. Bake until heated through, about 15 minutes. Serve crab cakes with sauce.

Serves 4. Per serving: 249 Calories; 49g Fat; 23g Protein; 12g Carbohydrate; 2g Dietary Fiber.

Avocado: *While recipes containing avocado may cause us to panic because of the high fat content we need not be overly concerned with avocado. The fat is oleic acid, a monounsaturated fat. It is believed to help lower LDL (bad) cholesterol and increase the health promoting HDL cholesterol. In addition, avocados are a good source of potassium, one of the electrolytes that help regulate blood pressure and guard against circulatory diseases such as high blood pressure, heart disease or stroke. Now, this is not to say we should eat a diet of all avocados all the time. But including moderate amounts of the fruit in our DIET is an intelligent choice.*

FISH TACOS IN ROMAINE LEAVES

Cheese is not typically served with fish; but if you like add a tablespoon or so of shredded cheese to your taco. Taco Toppings: diced fresh tomato, sliced green onions, chopped olives, sliced radishes, chopped avocado and shredded romaine all taste great on fish tacos.

Ingredients:
Cooking spray

4 (4-ounce) cod fillets, fresh or frozen

2 teaspoons low-sodium Mexican seasoning blend

¼-teaspoon salt

1 medium lime

1/2 cup sour cream, light

8 medium romaine lettuce leaves

Optional taco toppings: diced fresh tomato, sliced green onions, chopped olives, sliced radishes, chopped avocado and shredded romaine

Thaw fish, if frozen. Preheat broiler. Line broiler pan with heavy-duty aluminum foil and place rack on top. Spray liberally with cooking spray. In a small bowl combine the Mexican seasoning and salt. Rinse fish; pat dry with paper towels*. Season the fish with Mexican seasoning blend and salt mixture. Place the fish on the prepared broiler pan and cook under broiler for 4 to 6 minutes or until fish flakes easily when tested with a fork.

Meanwhile, finely shred enough peel from lime to make 1/2 teaspoon. Cut lime in half; squeeze enough juice to make 1 tablespoon. In a small bowl stir together the 1/2 teaspoon lime peel, the 1 tablespoon lime juice, and sour cream. Set aside.

Using a fork, flake fish into bite-size pieces. Divide fish among romaine leaves; roll up. Serve with sour cream mixture. Add taco toppings as desired.

Serves 4. Per serving: 111 Calories: 1g Fat; 21g Protein; 3g Carbohydrate; trace Dietary Fiber. *Patting the fish dry before cooking results in a crispy outer crust and a tender moist inner flesh.

GRILLED SALMON WITH CUCUMBER SALSA

The cool cucumber salsa flavored with fresh mint is the perfect complement to grilled salmon seasoned with lemon, salt and pepper. Enjoy fresh tossed greens dressed in vinegar and oil as a light and healthy side to this dish. Salmon is rich in omega-3 fatty acids which help lower triglycerides and may also fight cancer and reduce inflammation.

4 (6-ounce) salmon fillets, fresh or frozen

1 cup cucumber, seeded and chopped

2 Tablespoons green onions, sliced

2 Tablespoons white wine vinegar

2-teaspoons fresh mint leaves, chopped (or 1/2-teaspoon dried crushed mint leaves)

3-teaspoons olive oil, divided

1 Tablespoon lemon juice

Thaw fish, if frozen. For salsa, in a small bowl stir together cucumber, green onion, vinegar, mint leaves and 1 teaspoon olive oil. Cover and chill until ready to serve. Rinse fish; pat dry with paper towels. In a small bowl combine the remaining 2 teaspoons olive oil and lemon juice; brush over fish. Place fish on the greased rack of an uncovered grill directly over medium coals. Grill for 8 to 12 minutes or until fish flakes easily when tested with a fork, turning and brushing once with lemon mixture halfway through grilling. Serve salsa over fish.

Serves 4. Per serving: 234 Calories; 9g Fat; 34g Protein; 2g Carbohydrate; trace Dietary Fiber.

CREAMY CUCUMBER DRESSING

If you prefer a creamier dressing on your grilled salmon, try this recipe:

Combine 1 large cucumber, peeled and seeded with 1 cup sour cream light, 3 Tablespoons lemon juice, freshly squeezed, 1 bunch fresh dill, minced. Adjust seasoning with 1 Tablespoon sugar, 1/2 teaspoon salt, 1/8 teaspoon ground white pepper, a dash of Tabasco sauce. Mix well, spoon over grilled salmon.

PARMESAN BAKED FISH STICKS AND GARDEN PASTA SALAD

This is a kid friendly summer meal that is easy and healthy! WLS patients should eat pasta sparingly. Rely on the 2B/1B Rhythm and "Pasta as a Condiment" habits to ensure your enjoyment.

Parmesan Baked Fish Sticks

Cooking Spray

4 (4-ounce) cod fillets, thawed, cut into strips

1/4 cup Miracle Whip® light

2 Tablespoons Parmesan cheese, grated

1 Tablespoon fresh chives, snipped

1 teaspoon Worcestershire sauce

Preheat oven to 450°F. Spray a large rimmed baking sheet with cooking spray. In a small bowl stir together Miracle Whip® light, Parmesan cheese, chives, and Worcestershire sauce. Set aside. Rinse fish; pat dry with paper towels. Place fish on prepared baking sheet and spread Miracle Whip® light mixture evenly over fish. Bake uncovered in preheated oven for 12 to 15 minutes or until fish flakes easily when tested with a fork. Serve warm.

Serves 4. Per serving: 150 Calories; 5g Fat; 21g Protein; 3g Carbohydrate; trace Dietary Fiber.

SUMMERTIME GARDEN PASTA SALAD

Ingredients:

2 pounds firm, ripe, red tomatoes, washed, cored, diced

3 Tablespoons olive oil

16 large basil leaves, washed, torn into strips

Salt and freshly ground pepper

1 (10-ounce) package frozen peas

1 (8-ounce) package rotini pasta

2 Tablespoons butter

4 tablespoons freshly grated Parmesan cheese

Warm the olive oil in a large 12-inch skillet over medium heat. Add the diced tomato, half of the strips of basil, salt and pepper to taste. Cook and stir until thick sauce forms, about 20 minutes. Add the frozen peas and reduce heat to low while cooking pasta to package directions. Drain pasta and place in a large bowl, toss with butter. Add tomato sauce and toss. Sprinkle with Parmesan cheese. Serve warm with Parmesan Baked Fish Sticks.

Serves 6. Per serving: 315 Calories; 13g Fat; 10g Protein; 41g Carbohydrate; 5g Dietary Fiber.

While this recipe calls for halibut other firm flesh fish may be used; such as salmon, cod, shark, or swordfish. Shop the sale fliers and select the freshest fish available at your market. Halibut is a rich source of potassium containing 651mg per 4-ounce serving.

Ingredients:
Cooking spray
4 (4-ounce) halibut steaks
2 Tablespoons butter or margarine, softened
1 teaspoon *Provence herb blend
1 teaspoon lime peel, finely shredded
1 teaspoon lime juice
1 teaspoon butter or margarine, melted

For herb butter, in a small bowl stir together the 2 tablespoons softened butter, Provence herb blend, lime peel, and lime juice. Set aside.

Preheat broiler. Line broiler pan with heavy-duty aluminum foil and place rack on top. Spray liberally with cooking spray. Rinse halibut steaks; pat dry with paper towels. Place halibut on prepared rack of broiler pan. Brush with 1 teaspoon herb butter on each steak. Broil about 4 inches from the heat for 8 to 12 minutes or until fish flakes easily when tested with a fork, turning once halfway through broiling. Serve warm halibut with remaining herb butter.

Serves 4: Per serving: 185 Calories; 9g Fat; 24g Protein; trace Carbohydrate; trace Dietary Fiber.

*Provence herbs: While the thought of herbs de Provence evokes old world charm this seasoning mixture that usually contains savory, fennel, basil, thyme and lavender is actually as young as the 1970's. Typically Provence blends are used to flavor grilled foods such as this halibut dish. But the blend also serves to bring out the rich flavors of meat and vegetables in stews and in roasting. The ingredient that sets a Provence blend apart from other herb blends is lavender blossoms, which are pretty and aromatic. In addition, Provence blends do not contain sodium, spice or filler.

Seared Sea Scallops with Mushrooms & Pine Nuts

This quick skillet meal comes together in about 20 minutes.

Ingredients:
1/2 pound sea scallops, halved crosswise
¼-teaspoon salt
¼- teaspoon pepper
1 tablespoon unsalted butter
Cooking spray
2 cups sliced mushrooms
2 tablespoons pine nuts*, toasted
2 tablespoons minced shallots
1 garlic clove, minced
1/3 cup low sodium chicken broth
2 tablespoons fresh lemon juice
1 cup hot cooked angel hair (about 2 ounces uncooked pasta)

Season scallops with salt and pepper. Melt butter in a large 12-inch nonstick skillet coated with cooking spray over medium-high heat; add scallops, mushrooms, and pine nuts. Stir-fry 2 minutes or until scallops are done. Remove scallop mixture from skillet. Set aside; keep warm.

Add shallots and garlic to skillet; stir-fry 30 seconds. Stir in chicken broth and lemon juice. Bring to a boil; cook 2 minutes. Return scallop mixture to skillet; cook 30 seconds or until thoroughly heated. Serve over pasta.

Serves 2; Serving Size: 1 cup scallop mixture and 1/2 cup pasta. Per Serving: 337 Calories; 12g Fat; 28g Protein; 31g Carbohydrate; 3g Dietary Fiber.

*Pine nuts are the seeds found in pinecones. They may also be called pinon, pignoli and pignolia. At peak ripeness they have a delicate nutty flavor that is intensified with toasting. To toast: heat in a dry skillet over high heat, shaking the skillet constantly until the skin starts to brown and aroma is released. The high fat content of pine nuts will cause them to go rancid quickly: store refrigerated or frozen for up to 9 months.

Shrimp Louis Salad

This is the traditional Shrimp Louis salad made popular at the turn of the 20th Century. Don't feel bound by tradition: add fresh ingredients from your market for variety and nutrition. Chili sauce is found near the ketchup, mustard and barbecue sauce in your supermarket.

Ingredients:
4 cups iceberg lettuce, chopped (about ½ head)
1 large cucumber, sliced
2 large tomatoes, cut into wedges
2 eggs, hard-boiled, cut into wedges
1/2 cup olives
12 ounces shrimp, large, ready-to-eat
1 large lemon, cut into wedges
3 Tablespoons green onions, finely chopped
1½ cups Miracle Whip® light
1/4 cup chili sauce
1 Tablespoon lemon juice
1½-teaspoons Worcestershire sauce
¼-teaspoon hot pepper sauce

On each of four salad plates arrange the lettuce, cucumbers, tomatoes, eggs, olives and shrimp. Garnish with lemon wedges.

In a blender mince the green onions. Add the Miracle Whip® light, chili sauce, lemon juice, Worcestershire sauce and hot pepper sauce. Blend until smooth. Serve dressing on the side.

Serves 4. Per serving: 427 Calories; 29g Fat; 20g Protein; 24g Carbohydrate; 3g Dietary Fiber. "Louis" sauce is generally any mayonnaise-based sauce made with chili sauce and it is good with all manner of seafood and shellfish.

SHRIMP & MANGO WRAPS

For ease of preparation, use ready-to-eat shrimp found in the meat department or frozen food section of your supermarket. Look for low-carb wraps to increase your dietary fiber intake and reduce processed carbohydrate intake.

Dressing:
1/3 cup sour cream
1/3 cup Miracle Whip® light
1/4 cup basil, fresh, chopped

213

2 Tablespoons chives, chopped
1 teaspoon salt
¼-teaspoon black pepper
1 Tablespoon lemon juice, freshly squeezed

Salad:
1 1/2 pounds shrimp, peeled and deveined, ready-to-eat
1 large mango, peeled and cubed
4 (10-inch) flour tortillas
6 ounces lettuce leaves

Make dressing. Pulse sour cream, Miracle Whip Light, basil, chives, 1/2 teaspoon salt, and pepper in a blender until herbs are finely chopped and mixture is pale green. Stir-in lemon juice. Transfer dressing to a medium bowl. Coarsely chop shrimp; add to dressing along with mango and stir to combine.

Toast tortillas one at a time directly over burner at moderately high heat until puffed slightly and browned in spots but still flexible, 30 to 40 seconds. Transfer to a clean kitchen towel as toasted and stack, loosely wrapped in a towel.

Divide lettuce leaves among tortillas, arranging across the middle of each. Top with 1 1/4 cups shrimp salad. Tuck in ends of wraps, then roll up tightly to enclose filling. Cut wraps in half diagonally and serve.

Serves 4. Per serving: 573 Calories; 17g Fat; 42g Protein; 60g Carbohydrate; 5g Dietary Fiber.

Beef, Lamb, Pork

Beef is lean protein rich in iron and nutrients. It can also be stringy and difficult for some gastric bypass patients to digest because we lack the necessary enzymes needed to adequately break down the protein for digestion. Before advancing protein back into our post-WLS it is important to consult with our bariatric centers for advice.

Once given the go-ahead many of us do enjoy beef as part of our DAY 6 DIET. Beef is a great source of iron at 17% our Daily Value in a 3-ounce serving. That serving provides 184 Calories and 30g Protein with 6g Fat (2 Saturated) 77mg Cholesterol; and 38mg Sodium. It is rich in vitamin B12; zinc; niacin; riboflavin; and B6.

Easy Beef Stroganoff

Stroganoff is named after the 19th-century Russian diplomat Count Paul Stroganov. It is a dish of thin slices of beef quickly cooked with sliced onions and mushrooms in butter and finished with sour cream. In the United States we serve it over egg noodles. Remember our DAY 6 DIET Intelligent Basics from Part 2 and use the starchy noodles as a condiment to avoid overeating.

Ingredients:
2 cups egg noodles, yolk-free, uncooked
1 pound beef round
4 teaspoons canola oil
¼-teaspoon salt
¼-teaspoon pepper
1 clove garlic, minced

1 package (8-ounces) mushrooms, sliced
1 package brown gravy mix
1 cup cold water
1/4 cup sour cream, light

Prepare egg noodles according to package directions and keep warm. Cut beef round against the grain into 1/4-inch thick strips. Heat 2 teaspoons of canola oil in a large 12-inch skillet over medium-high heat. Add 1/2 of beef and cook and stir for one minute or until outside surface of beef is no longer pink. Do not overcook. Remove from skillet to a platter and tent with aluminum foil. Add remaining 2 teaspoons vegetable oil and cook remaining beef. Transfer second batch of beef to plate and season with salt and pepper. Tent with foil.

In same skillet cook garlic and mushrooms until tender and aromatic. Add gravy mix and 1 cup of cold water to skillet, stirring constantly until gravy thickens. Remove from heat and stir in sour cream. Add beef to gravy and stir to coat.

Serve stroganoff with warm egg noodles, 1/2 cup of noodles per normal serving, 1-2 Tablespoons WLS serving.

Serves 4. Per Serving: 377 Calories; 20g Fat; 28g Protein; 20g Carbohydrate; 2g Dietary Fiber.

SALISBURY STEAK WITH MUSHROOM GRAVY

I have never overcome my love of Salisbury Steak. Today this continues to be a standby for me and I use all matter of ground meat including ground wild game meat. Using prepared gravy simplifies things, and as always, leftovers are wonderful! Traditionally Salisbury Steak is served with mashed potatoes, but I find steamed vegetables such as green beans or carrots are just as complimentary without the heaviness of starch.

Ingredients:
16-ounces lean ground beef, lean
1/3 cup onion, finely chopped
1/4 cup saltine crackers, crumbled

1 egg white, slightly beaten

2 tablespoons milk

1 tablespoon prepared cream-style horseradish

¼-teaspoon salt

1/8-teaspoon pepper

1 (12-ounce) jar brown beef gravy

4 ounces fresh mushrooms, sliced

2 tablespoons reduced sodium beef broth

In a medium bowl combine the ground beef, onion, saltine cracker crumbs, egg white, milk, horseradish, salt and pepper. Shape into four 1/2-inch thick patties.

Heat large 12-inch nonstick skillet over medium heat until hot. Place beef patties in skillet; cook 7 to 8 minutes or until no longer pink and juices run clear, turning once. Remove from skillet; keep warm.

In same skillet, combine gravy, mushrooms and reduced sodium beef broth. Simmer over medium heat 3 to 5 minutes or until mushrooms are tender. Serve over Salisbury steak.

Serves 4. Per serving: 411 Calories; 26g Fat; 24g Protein; 18g Carbohydrate; 1g Dietary Fiber.

Substitution Hint: If you prefer, substitute ground turkey or ground chicken for the ground beef but add an extra egg white to ensure your steaks are moist and tender.

OVEN BAKED PORCUPINE MEATBALLS

This recipe reminds me of the great casserole foods from the 1970's. My mom made the meatballs with the rice mixed in with the meat. But rolling the meatballs in the pre-soaked rice gives the meatballs more bite without overindulgence in starchy carbohydrate. Any ground meat will work in this recipe, but if you use ground chicken or turkey be sure to add a small amount of olive oil or other fat so the meatballs are succulent.

Ingredients:

1 cup white rice

Cooking spray

1 pound ground veal
1 Tablespoon rice wine vinegar
1 bunch green onions, minced
1/2 cup water chestnuts*, canned, drained, diced
1 Tablespoon cornstarch
1 egg white, lightly beaten
1 teaspoon sugar
½-teaspoon sesame oil
1 teaspoon salt
¼-teaspoon white pepper

Soak rice in hot tap water in a large bowl while preparing meat mixture. Line a large baking sheet with foil and place baking rack on top so that fat will drip through rack to foil lined sheet. Spray rack with cooking spray. Set aside.

Preheat oven to 350°F.Combine ground veal, rice wine vinegar, green onions, diced water chestnuts, cornstarch, egg white, sugar, sesame oil, salt and pepper. Mix well. Form into 24 evenly sized meatballs. Drain rice in a sieve and transfer to a shallow dish. Roll each meatball in rice to coat and place 1-inch apart on baking rack. Bake in preheated oven for 18-22 minutes or until meatballs are done. Serve warm.

Serves 6, 4 meatballs each. Per serving:243 Calories; 6g Fat; 18g Protein; 28g Carbohydrate; 1g Dietary Fiber.

Water chestnuts are the edible tuber of a water plant found in Southeast Asia. They are bland with a hint of sweetness and valued for the crunch they add to stir-fried dishes.

RED CURRY BEEF AND PEPPERS

This is a showy basic beef curry recipe. Change it up by adding different vegetables such as broccoli, onions, mushrooms or bamboo shoots. Curry is often served over rice, but it is equally good without any starchy accompaniment, which may cause pouch discomfort while providing little nutritional value. Try this recipe with chicken tenders, pork, or even firm tofu in place of the beef.

Ingredients:

16-ounces beef round, thinly sliced

1 Tablespoon canola oil

1 Tablespoon curry paste, red

2 medium bell peppers cut into strips

1 Tablespoon fish sauce

1 teaspoon sugar

Soy sauce, low sodium

Cut beef into strips and set aside. In a large 12-inch skillet heat oil over medium high heat. Add red curry paste and cook and stir briefly to soften and blend. And beef and cook and stir for 3 to 5 minutes until done. Add bell peppers, fish sauce and sugar. Cook and stir for three minutes or until peppers are soft. Serve hot with reduced sodium soy sauce.

Serves 4. Per serving: 310 Calories; 21g Fat; 24g Protein; 6g Carbohydrate; 1g Dietary Fiber.

TOMATO BASIL CURRY

If you don't care for bell peppers, try this quick beef curry. In a large 12-inch skillet heat 1 tablespoon vegetable oil and 1 tablespoon red curry paste. Add 1-pound beef round, thinly sliced and cook and stir until beef is cooked through. Add 1 medium tomato, diced, and 1 can low-fat coconut milk. Simmer five minutes, stirring twice. Stir in a handful of chopped fresh basil and serve warm.

MOJO BEEF KABOBS

Mojo sauce originated in the Canary Islands and is popular in Cuban and Caribbean cuisine. Home cooks in these regions specialize in the sauce, which usually includes citrus juice, vinegar and seasonings of garlic, paprika, and cumin. It is becoming increasingly popular in the United States particularly the Southern foodie states of Florida, Texas and Louisiana.

Ingredients:

1/4 cup orange juice

1/4 cup lime juice

3 Tablespoons oregano, finely chopped
3 Tablespoons olive oil
2 Tablespoons parsley, finely chopped
1 teaspoon ground cumin
1 teaspoon garlic, minced
¾-teaspoon salt
16 ounces beef sirloin, cut 1-inch thick
1 teaspoon black pepper
1 large lime, cut into wedges
1 small red onion, cut into wedges
1-pint cherry tomatoes

For Mojo Sauce: Whisk together orange juice, lime juice, oregano, olive oil, parsley, cumin, garlic, and salt. Set aside. Cut beef steak into 1 1/4-inch pieces: season with pepper. Alternately thread beef with lime and onion wedges evenly onto four 12-inch metal skewers. Thread tomatoes evenly onto four 12-inch metal skewers.

Place kabobs on grid over medium, ash-covered coals. Grill tomato kabobs, uncovered, about 2 to 4 minutes or until slightly softened, turning occasionally. Grill beef kabobs, uncovered, about 8 to 10-minutes for medium-rare to medium doneness, turning occasionally Serve kabobs drizzled with mojo sauce.

Serves 4. Per serving: 386 Calories; 27g Fat; 23g Protein; 15g Carbohydrate; 3g Dietary Fiber.

HERBED LAMB MEATBALLS AND GREEK SALAD

Ground lamb is particularly tender and lends itself to tasty meatballs. These no-mess treats are baked in the oven to avoid stove frying and splatter. Enjoy with this nutrient dense Greek Salad.

Ingredients:
1 1/2 pounds lean ground lamb
1/2 cup dry bread crumbs
1/2 cup (2 ounces) crumbled feta cheese
3 tablespoons chopped fresh parsley

1 teaspoon dried mint flakes
¼-teaspoon salt
¼-teaspoon pepper
2 garlic cloves, crushed
Cooking spray

Preheat oven to 400º. Combine all ingredients except cooking spray in a large bowl and stir well. Shape mixture into 30 (1 1/2-inch) meatballs. Place meatballs on a broiler pan coated with cooking spray. Bake for 15 minutes or until meatballs are done. While meatballs bake make Greek Salad.

Serves 6. Per serving: 391 Calories; 30g Fat; 22g Protein; 8g Carbohydrate; trace Dietary Fiber.

GREEK SALAD

Ingredients:
1 cup diced seeded peeled cucumber
1 cup diced red bell pepper
1 cup diced green bell pepper
1/2 cup (2 ounces) crumbled Feta cheese
1/4 cup diced red onion
1/4 cup chopped pepperoncini peppers
1/4 cup kalamata olives, pitted and chopped
2 tablespoons lemon juice
2 teaspoons dried oregano
1 teaspoon extra-virgin olive oil
¼-teaspoon ground white pepper

Toss all ingredients in a bowl. Serve with baked meatballs.

Serves 6. Per serving: 89 Calories; 6g Fat; 2g Protein; 7g Carbohydrate; 2g Dietary Fiber.

LAMB CASSOULET

I have truly grown to adore the flavor of lamb and this cassoulet makes the most of tender lamb shoulder. Once the ingredients are together in a large Dutch oven the work is done. All you need do is sit back and anticipate the delicious meal to come.

Ingredients:

2 slices lean bacon, chopped

2 tablespoons olive oil

1 pound-boneless lamb shoulder, cut into 1-inch pieces

1/2 pound-Polish smoked sausage, sliced into 1-inch pieces

1 1/2 cups chopped onion

½-teaspoon salt

1 (28-ounce) can diced tomatoes with juice

2 cloves garlic, finely chopped

1 celery stalk, sliced

1 leek, sliced (white part only)

1 tablespoon chopped parsley

½-teaspoon dried thyme

¼-teaspoon pepper

2 (15-ounce) cans white beans, rinsed and drained

Preheat oven to 350°F. In large oven proof Dutch oven over medium-high heat, cook bacon until crisp. Drain and crumble; set aside. In the same Dutch oven, heat oil over medium-high heat. Add lamb and sausage; cook until browned. Add onion and salt; cook 3 minutes. Stir in bacon, tomatoes, garlic, celery, leek, parsley, thyme and pepper. Bring to a boil. Stir in beans. Bake in preheated oven for 90 minutes or until lamb is tender. Ladle into bowls and serve warm.

Serves 8. Per serving: 414 Calories; 22g Fat; 21g Protein; 33g Carbohydrate; 7g Dietary Fiber.

ITALIAN PORK SKILLET WITH EGGPLANT & SQUASH

This is a great skillet meal particularly if carb cravings have you in a cranky mood. The meal is rich in heart-healthy complex carbohydrates that tame the Carb Monster and provide the nutrients your body needs to build a strong immune system. And it comes together in short order. Be sure and save leftovers for lunch the next day.

Ingredients:

1 pound pork tenderloin

1 small eggplant

1 medium summer squash

2 tablespoons olive oil, divided
¾-teaspoon salt
¼-teaspoon pepper
1 clove garlic, minced
1 medium onion, thinly sliced
1 small red pepper, cut into thin strips
1 teaspoon Italian seasoning blend
¾-teaspoon salt
1/3 cup water
1 teaspoon cornstarch

Partially freeze tenderloin; cut pork diagonally into 1/4-inch thick slices; quarter the slices. Cut squash lengthwise in half. Place on flat sides and cut crosswise into 1/4-inch-thick slices. In a skillet, brown half the pork in 1 tablespoon hot olive oil, stirring constantly; remove from pan.

Add the remaining pork; cook, stirring constantly till pork is browned. Sprinkle 3/4 teaspoon salt and the pepper over pork. Place the remaining olive oil, eggplant and minced garlic in skillet and cook over medium-high heat for 3 minutes.

Add squash, onion, red pepper, Italian seasoning blend, and 3/4 teaspoon salt; cook for 7 minutes, stirring occasionally. Combine water and cornstarch; stir into vegetables. Return pork to skillet and cook for 3-4 minutes or till thickened, stirring occasionally. Serve warm, like a thick stew.

Serves 4. Per serving: 258 Calories; 11g Fat; 26g Protein; 14g Carbohydrate; 5g Dietary Fiber.

CALYPSO PORK CHOPS

Ingredients:
4 (6-ounce) boneless pork loin chops
1 cup chicken broth
1/2 cup orange juice
2 tablespoons dark rum (optional)
2 tablespoons lime juice

2 tablespoons brown sugar
1 clove garlic, minced
½-teaspoon salt
½-teaspoon ground ginger
¼-teaspoon ground nutmeg
¼-teaspoon ground cloves

Combine all ingredients in a resealable plastic bag; seal bag and refrigerate for 4-24 hours. Preheat grill or broiler to medium-high heat. Remove chops from marinade; discard leftover marinade. Grill chops quickly over indirect heat in covered grill about 10-12 minutes, turning once to brown both sides. Serve warm with Honey-Grilled Vegetables.

Serves 4. Per serving: 249 Calories; 10g Fat; 30g Protein; 6g Carbohydrate; trace Dietary Fiber.

HONEY-GRILLED VEGETABLES

12 small red potatoes, halved
1/4 cup honey
3 tablespoons dry white wine
1 clove garlic, minced
1 teaspoon crushed dried thyme leaves
½-teaspoon salt
½-teaspoon pepper
2 zucchinis, halved lengthwise
1 medium eggplant, cut into 1/2-inch-thick slices
1 green bell pepper, halved
1 red bell pepper, halved
1 large onion, cut into wedges

Cover potatoes with water in large saucepan. Bring to a boil over medium-high heat. Cook 5 minutes; drain. Combine honey, wine, garlic, thyme, salt and pepper in small bowl; mix well. Place potatoes and remaining vegetables on oiled barbecue grill over hot coals. Grill 20 to 25 minutes, turning and brushing with honey mixture every 7 to 8 minutes.

Serves 4. Per serving: 322 Calories; 1g Fat; 8g Protein; 10g Dietary Fiber.

SOUTHWESTERN GRILLED PORK TENDERLOIN WITH TOMATO & BASIL SALAD

Tenderloin is my favorite cut of pork. It is juicy, lean, and remarkably easy to prepare. I found this recipe from the National Pork Producers Council and have not been compelled to change a thing.

Ingredients:
2 (12-ounce) pork tenderloins, unseasoned
5 teaspoons chili powder
1½-teaspoons dried oregano
¾-teaspoon ground cumin
2 garlic cloves, minced
1 tablespoon vegetable oil

In a small bowl, mix well all seasonings and vegetable oil. Rub mixture over all surfaces of tenderloins. Cover and refrigerate 2-24 hours. Grill over medium-hot coals, turning occasionally, for 15-20 minutes, until thermometer inserted reads 155-160ºF. Pork is done when there is still a hint of pink in the center. Slice to serve.

Serves 6. Per serving: 166 Calories; 7g Fat; 24g Protein; 2g Carbohydrate; 1g Dietary Fiber.

MARINATED TOMATO-BASIL SALAD

Ingredients:
32 slices (1/2-inch-thick) red tomato (about 8 tomatoes or 4 1/4 pounds)
1 cup thinly sliced red onion, separated into rings
1/2 cup chopped fresh basil
1/2 cup rice vinegar
1 tablespoon olive oil
1 teaspoon sugar
½-teaspoon salt

Arrange tomato slices and onion in a 13 × 9-inch dish. Combine basil and remaining ingredients and stir well with a whisk. Pour over tomatoes and onion. Cover and chill at least 2 hours.

Serving Size: 4 tomato slices. Per serving: 42 Calories; 2g Fat; 1g Protein; 6g Carbohydrate; 1g Dietary Fiber.

FRUIT DESSERTS

Years ago, during year four post-op I went through a phase of fake desserts. By that I mean sugar free cakes with fat free sugar free topping and all kinds of fake ingredients that masqueraded as traditional sweet sticky carbohydrate thick desserts. They did taste good. But then I started doing a bit of research and it turns out all those fake ingredients were simply chemically altered mutations of the things (sugar and trans-fat) that I should not be eating in the first place. No wonder even the fake desserts were leaving me in a food coma stupor.

Earlier in Part I we talked about the freedom that surrender brings. For me there was nothing more liberating than surrendering to the fact that sweet carbohydrate heavy desserts were no longer an option in my diet. It is just a matter of fact. It is just a way of life: I don't have to play the fake dessert game any longer.

This liberation led me to the discovery of fruit for dessert: a completely new and foreign concept to me. Fruit desserts are easy to prepare, they are loaded with vitamins, antioxidants and fiber. They are naturally sweet and pretty. They put the intelligent in our DAY 6 DIET! Here you will find several fruit dessert recipes here and I hope you will enjoy them as much as I do.

STRAWBERRIES ROMANOFF

This lovely dessert may also be served as a breakfast treat, but make sure you have protein first (Rule #1) and omit the strawberry liqueur. (Hint: Increase the protein by adding a scoop of unflavored protein powder to the yogurt; stir until dissolved) If strawberries are out of season use other fresh fruit or berries as desired.

Ingredients:
1 cup plain non-fat yogurt
1/4 cup firmly packed brown sugar or brown sugar substitute
½-teaspoon ground cinnamon
1 teaspoon vanilla extract
2 tablespoons strawberry liqueur (optional)
2 pints fresh strawberries, hulled, and cut in bite-sized pieces
2 tablespoons pecans, chopped, lightly toasted, for garnish

In a small bowl, whisk yogurt, brown sugar, cinnamon, vanilla extract, and strawberry liqueur until fully mixed. Refrigerate for at least 1 hour to make the sauce slightly firm. Divide berries evenly into four dessert dishes. Spoon 1/4 cup sauce over each serving. Top with nuts and serve immediately.

Serves 4. Per serving: 111 Calories; 2g Fat; 4g Protein; 16g Carbohydrate; 1g Dietary Fiber.

French chefs created the deliciously decadent Romanoff desserts for the Russian royal family of the same name. In some variations the berries are soaked in orange juice or Cointreau and then topped with whipped cream.

PEACHES IN RED WINE & SOUR CREAM TOPPING

This is an elegant finish to a fine autumnal meal. The wine reduction should be prepared the day before serving and the peaches set to soak early in the day of the meal. Serve the peaches in shallow bowls for a dramatic presentation and sprinkle the sour cream topping lightly with cinnamon for garnish.

Ingredients:
1/4 cup sugar
1/4 cup orange rind strips (about 1 orange)
1/4 cup lemon rind strips (about 2 large lemons)
1/8 teaspoon ground cardamom
7 whole cloves
4 black peppercorns
1 (3-inch) cinnamon stick

1 (750-milliliter) bottle dry red wine
6 cups fresh sliced peaches (about 2 1/4 pounds)
1-pint sour cream
2 teaspoons granulated sugar
Ground cinnamon for garnish.

In a large, 2-quart saucepot bring sugar, orange rind, lemon rind, ground cardamom, cloves, peppercorns, cinnamon stick and dry red wine to a boil over medium-high heat. Reduce heat and cook 10 minutes or until wine mixture is reduced to 1 1/2 cups. Cool to room temperature. May be prepared the day before.

Strain wine mixture through a sieve over a bowl, and discard solids. Combine wine mixture and peaches in a medium bowl; cover and chill 4 hours, stirring occasionally.

In a small bowl combine sour cream and 2 teaspoons granulated sugar, stirring until sugar dissolves. Divide peaches among six shallow dessert bowls and top each with 1 tablespoon of sour cream topping. Sprinkle with ground cinnamon.

Serves 6. Per serving: 227 Calories; 4g Fat; 3g Protein; 36g Carbohydrate; 7g Dietary Fiber.

SUMMER FRUIT WITH SPARKLING CUSTARD SAUCE

Nectarines and raspberries are so lovely together. Adding a dollop of sparkling custard sauce turns an ordinary bowl of fruit into a celebration. The custard may be prepared the day before to the point of covering and chilling. Stir in the sparkling wine just before serving.

1 1/4 cups 1% low-fat milk
1/2 cup sugar
1 tablespoon cornstarch
1 large egg, lightly beaten
1 teaspoon vanilla extract
3/4 cup sparkling wine or club soda
1 1/2 cups fresh raspberries
3 medium nectarines, each cut into 8 wedges

Heat milk over medium-high heat in a heavy saucepan to 180ºF or until tiny bubbles form around edge (do not boil). Remove from heat.

Combine sugar and cornstarch in a medium heavy saucepan; add milk, stirring with a whisk. Cook over medium heat 4 minutes or until thick, stirring constantly. Gradually add hot milk mixture to egg in a bowl, stirring constantly with a whisk. Return milk mixture to pan. Cook over medium-low heat 6 minutes or until thick, stirring constantly. Remove from heat. Pour into a bowl; stir in vanilla. Cover surface with plastic wrap; chill.

Stir sparkling wine or club soda into chilled custard and serve with raspberries and nectarines.

Serving Size: 1/3 cup custard sauce, 1/4 cup berries, and 4 nectarine slices. Per serving: 179 Calories; 2g Fat; 4g Protein; 33g Carbohydrate; 3g Dietary Fiber.

WARM BAKED PEACHES OR NECTARINES

Although this recipe calls for peaches or nectarines, any stone fruit will work. In fact, a variety of stone fruit such as peaches, plums, apricots, and nectarines would make a lovely dish for a family dinner or potluck. Use the best seasonally fresh fruit available to you and follow the method as described below.

4 freestone peaches or nectarines

1 lemon

1 vanilla bean

2 Tablespoons granulated sugar

2 Tablespoons unsalted butter

Preheat oven to 350°F. Cut the peaches or the nectarines in half. Remove the pits. Place them, cut side up in a well-buttered ovenproof baking dish. Split the vanilla bean and scrape the seeds into the sugar. Sprinkle the fruit with the sugar and lemon juice. Place a small piece of the butter in the center of each half fruit and bake at 350°F until tender and lightly browned, for approximately 20 minutes. Serve warm.

Serves 8. Per serving: 101 Calories; 6g Fat; trace Protein; 13g Carbohydrate; 1g Dietary Fiber.

Brandied Apples and Pears

Serve with a dollop of low-fat vanilla yogurt.

2 peeled Bosc pears, cored and quartered

2 peeled Golden Delicious apples, cored and quartered

2 peeled Rome apples, cored and quartered

1/4 cup golden raisins

1 teaspoon ground cinnamon

1/4 cup apricot preserves

1/4 cup apple juice

3 tablespoons Calvados (apple brandy)

Combine all ingredients in a heavy saucepan; cook over low heat 30 minutes or until fruit is soft, stirring occasionally. Serving Size: 1/2 cup. Per serving: 116 Calories; trace Fat; trace Protein; 27g Carbohydrate; 3g Dietary Fiber.

Layered Fruit Salad

This is a lovely brunch side dish or dessert. If you prefer use 1/3 fat cream cheese. You may also toss all the fruit together in the bowl and serve the topping in a separate bowl so individuals may select how much topping they wish to include with their fruit. If melons are in season, they make a nice addition to the salad.

2 cups fresh or frozen peaches

2 cups fresh blueberries

2 cups fresh strawberry slices

2 cups fresh green grapes

2 tablespoons lemon juice

1 tablespoon grated lemon rind

8 ounces cream cheese, softened

1 cup whipping cream

1/4 cup powdered sugar

1/2 cup walnuts, chopped

In a large glass trifle bowl layer peaches, blueberries, strawberries and green grapes, arranging the layers so they look pretty from the outside of the bowl.

231

In a large mixing bowl using an electric mixer beat together the lemon juice, lemon rind, and softened cream cheese, until smooth.

In another bowl beat the whipping cream until peaks form. Slowly add the powdered sugar, whipping until soft peaks form. Fold the whipped cream mixture into the cream cheese mixture and gently combine. Spread over the layered fruit. Top with the chopped walnuts. Serve immediately.

Serves 16. Per serving: 166 Calories; 13g Fat; 3g Protein; 12g Carbohydrate; 2g Dietary Fiber.

CRANBERRY POACHED PEARS

This is one of my favorite winter holiday desserts. It is unusually rich for a fruit dessert and beautifully finishes an elegant holiday menu. I have used light cranberry juice cocktail with good results.

3 large pears
2 cups cranberry juice cocktail
1/4 cup firmly packed brown sugar
1 teaspoon whole cloves
1 (3-inch) cinnamon stick
3 tablespoons low-fat sour cream
ground cinnamon, for garnish

Peel and core pears. Cut each pear in half lengthwise; set aside. Combine juice, brown sugar, cloves, and cinnamon in a large non-aluminum saucepot; bring to a boil. Place pears cut sides up, in a single layer in pan; cover, reduce heat, and simmer 8 minutes or until pears are tender. Remove from heat. Let stand, covered, 20 minutes. Remove pears with a slotted spoon, and place in a shallow dish. Cover and chill.

Bring juice mixture to a boil; cook 5 minutes or until reduced to 1 cup. Strain juice mixture through a sieve into a small bowl; cover and chill. Discard spices.

Arrange 1 pear half; cut side up, on each of 6 dessert plates. Drizzle 2 1/2 tablespoons juice mixture over each pear half; top each with 1 1/2 teaspoons sour cream. Garnish with a sprinkle of ground cinnamon.

Serves: 6. Per serving: 142 Calories; 1g Fat; 1g Protein; 35g Carbohydrate; 2g Dietary Fiber.

CONDIMENTS

This is your opportunity for culinary creativity. I invite you to look beyond the ketchup and mustard bottle and discover a world of fascinating flavors and textures in the condiment aisle. Think sweet and savory and both at the same time. The more complex the flavor combination the happier your palate will be and the less likely you will experience post-meal cravings.

Shop for unusual condiments at World Market, Whole Foods, boutique style gift shops, the farmer's markets and local craft fairs. Many regional artisans are thriving in the trade of locally grown produce crafted into fine condiments sold at homespun stands and fair booths.

At first glance $5.75 for a jar of handcrafted sauce may seem alarming. But if you consider that each 1-pint jar of sauce contains 32 servings you are spending only .18 cents per serving to please your palate with something different and delicious.

Use your average grilled baked or poached protein as a pallet of discovery on your tour of world condiments. And don't forget to give these easy fail-proof recipes a try.

COMPOUND BUTTERS

Compound butters are easy to prepare considering the flavor payoff you receive. Simply by adding a few well-chosen ingredients to room temperature butter we can easily create a condiment that takes an ordinary piece of protein beyond the extraordinary. Here are a few of my favorite flavor combinations. Using seasonal herbs keeps flavors interesting and your palate never need be bored again. In addition, the inclusion of a small amount of fat (1 teaspoon to 3 ounces lean protein) creates a coating on the tongue called mouth feel that lends to your overall culinary experience. In other words, your mind registers satiation more than it would with a plain piece of lean protein.

Ingredients:
1/4-pound unsalted butter, room temperature

Choice of ingredients, below

Seasoned Compound Butter: To the butter add 1 Tablespoon all-purpose seasoning.

Herb Butter: To the butter add 1-2 Tablespoons fresh minced herbs.

Honey-Mustard: To the butter add 1 Tablespoon fresh unfiltered honey and 1 teaspoon dry mustard.

Louisiana Butter: To the butter add 1 teaspoon Old Bay Seafood Seasoning and 2-3 dashes of Louisiana Hot Sauce.

Garlic-Herb Butter: To the butter add 1 clove minced garlic and 1 teaspoon minced fresh herbs.

Blue Cheese Butter: To the butter add 1-ounce crumbled blue cheese.

Chipotle Butter: To the butter add 1 chopped chipotle pepper.

For each variation above, blend butter and ingredients together with a wooden spoon. Spoon mixture onto parchment paper and form into a log about 1-inch diameter. Roll tightly and seal ends. Wrap in plastic wrap. Refrigerate until use. 1 teaspoon per 3-ounces of protein is a serving.

Per 1 teaspoon compound butter: 34 Calories; 4g Fat; trace other nutrients.

GARLIC JELLY

This may sound strange at first but when used in small amounts to moisten and season lean protein this jelly packs a powerful flavor punch. The slightly sweet garlicky condiment is good whisked into soups, gravies and sauces.

One batch makes three half pints which store well refrigerated. Don't be afraid of the sugar in this recipe because it is enjoyed in such small quantities with protein that your blood sugar will not be adversely affected. In addition, enjoying a slightly sweet flavor with lean protein tends to increase the length of time we experience satiation.

Ingredients:
3 cups white wine vinegar
1/2 cup garlic, peeled and chopped
6 cups sugar
2 cups water
6 ounces liquid pectin

In a 2½-quart saucepan, simmer the vinegar and garlic for about 15 minutes. Remove the pan from the heat and cool slightly. Pour the liquid into a clean 1-quart glass jar. Cover the jar and let stand at room temperature for 24 - 48 hours.

Strain the vinegar and garlic through a wire strainer into a 6-quart kettle. Discard garlic. Measure 2 cups of liquid. Add more uncooked white wine vinegar, if necessary, to equal two cups. Add the sugar and water to the vinegar, stirring to dissolve the sugar. Bring to a full rolling boil over high heat.

Stir in the liquid pectin and return the mixture to a boil for exactly 1 minute, stirring constantly. Skim off any foam with a metal spoon. Pour the jelly into hot, clean jars, leaving 1/4 inch of headspace. Cap and seal. Process in a boiling-water-bath canner for 10 minutes.

PEPPER & PAPAYA RELISH

This relish is particularly delicious served over skillet cooked fresh fish or pork. While protein rests on a plate warm the relish in the cooking skillet and serve atop fish or pork. May also be served chilled over crisp greens for a refreshing salad dressing. One serving is about 1/3 cup. For convenience use bottled roasted red peppers, canned roasted green chilies and canned diced papaya that is preserved in natural juice without added sugar.

Ingredients:
2 roasted red peppers, diced
3 papayas, seeded and diced
3 roasted green chilies, seeded and diced
1 red onion, diced
1 lime, juiced
1 Tablespoon rice vinegar
1 Tablespoon honey
Salt and pepper, to taste

In a large bowl, stir together diced roasted red peppers, diced papayas, roasted green chilies, diced red onions, lime juice, rice vinegar, honey and salt and pepper to taste. Allow to stand at room temperature for flavors to marry. Store unused relish in refrigerator. Use within one week.

SLADE'S COCKTAIL SAUCE

Slade is my stepson and he makes an outstanding cocktail sauce that we enjoy at our family dinners with chilled ready-to-eat shrimp. He uses Heinz ketchup but if you are watching your sugar calories low-carbohydrate ketchup may be used with favorable results. This sauce is also good served with traditional Maryland crab cakes.

Ingredients:
1/3 cup horseradish sauce, creamy style
1 cup ketchup
1 medium lemon, zested and juiced
Salt and pepper

Combine horseradish sauce, ketchup, lemon zest and lemon juice in a small bowl stirring well to combine. Taste and season with salt and pepper to taste. Add additional horseradish to taste. Keep chilled until serving with peeled ready-to-eat shrimp.

THAI VEGETABLE RELISH

Garlic chili pepper sauce can be found in the Asian food section of most supermarkets.

Ingredients:
1 large tomato
1/2 medium red bell pepper
2 chili peppers, minced
1/4 cup basil, fresh, chopped
2 cloves garlic, minced
2 Tablespoons cider vinegar
1 Tablespoon fish sauce
garlic chili pepper sauce, to taste

In a medium bowl combine tomato, red bell pepper, chili peppers, basil, garlic, cider vinegar, fish sauce. Season with garlic chili pepper sauce to taste. Serve at room temperature.

BIBLIOGRAPHY

Agatston, Arthur MD. The South Beach Diet: A Doctor's Plan for Fast and Lasting Weight Loss. Headline Book Publishing, London.

Agatston, Arthur MD. The South Beach Diet: Dining Guide.Rodale, Birmingham, AL.

Bailey, Kaye (Editor). A Collection of Neighborhood Recipes: LivingAfterWLS a safe haven circle of friends. Morris Press Cookbooks, Kearney, NE.

Bailey, Kaye. The 5 Day Pouch Test Owner's Manual. LivingAfterWLS, LLC. Morris Printing, Kearney, NE.

Baker, Dan PhD., Stauth, Cameron. What Happy People Know. Rodale, United States.

Beard, Lina and Beard, Adelia Belle, The Original Girl's Handy Book. Black Dog & Leventhal Publishers Inc., New York, NY

Better Homes & Gardens. 15 Minutes or Less Low-Carb Recipes. Meridith Books, Des Moines, Iowa.

Better Homes & Gardens. The Smart Diet: The right approach to weight loss. Meridith Books, Des Moines, Iowa.

Brand-Miller, Jennie MD, Wolever, Thomas M.S. MD, Foster-Powell, Kaye, Colagiuri, Stephen, MD. The New Glucose Revolution: The Authoritative Guide to The Glycemic Index - the Dietary Solution for Lifelong Health. Marlowe & Company, New York, NY.

Breathnach, Sarah Ban, The Simple Abundance Companion. Warner Books, New York, NY.

Cooking Light, 5 Ingredient, 15 Minute Cookbook. Oxmoor House, Birmingham, AL.

Cooking Light, Superfast Suppers: Speedy Solutions for Dinner Dilemmas. Oxmoor House, Birmingham, AL.

Culpepper, Mary Kay (Editor). Cooking Light Magazine. Birmingham, AL.

Eades, Michael R. MD, Eades, Mary Dan MD. Protein Power: The High-Protein/Low-Carbohydrate Way to Lose Weight, Feel Fit, and Boost Your Health - in Just Weeks! Bantam Books, New York, NY.

Havala, Suzanne M.S., R.D. Being Vegetarian for Dummies. Wiley Publishing, Nic. Hoboken, NJ.

Jensen, Bernard MD. Guide to Body Chemistry & Nurtirion. Keats Publishing, Los Angeles, CA.

Johnson, Kristina M. (Editor-in-Chief). Women's Health. Rodale, Emmaus, PA.

Ketcham, Katherine, Asbury, William F. Beyond the Influence: Understanding and Defeating Alcoholism. Bantom Book. United States.

Latona, Valerie (Editor In Chief). Shape Magazine. United States.

Litin, Scott C. MD (Editor in Chief). Mayo Clinic Family Health Book. HarperResource, New York, NY.

Marber, Ian and Edgson, Vicki; The Food Doctor: Healing foods for mind and body. Collins & Brown Ltd., London.

Martha Stewart's Hors D'Oeuvres Handbook. Clarkson Potter, New York.

Natow, Annette B.; Heslin PhD., RD, Jo-Ann M.A., R.D. The Protein Counter, 2nd Edition. Pocket Books, New York, NY.

Ostman, Barbara Gibbs; Baker, Jane L. The Recipe Writer's Handbook. John Wiley & Sons, Inc., Hoboken, NJ.

Reader's Digest, Eat Well Stay Well. Reader's Digest Association, Inc. Pleasantville, NY.

Rewega, Alicia (Editor). Clean Eating. Mississauga, Ontario, Canada.

Smith, Art. Back to the Table; The Reunion of Food and Family. Hyperion: New York. 2001.

Swilley, Dana RD. UCLA Division of General Surgery, Section of Minimally Invasive and Bariatric Surgery. "Micronutrient and Macronutrient Needs in Roux-en-Y Gastric Bypass Patients. March 2008. Bariatric Times.

The Best of Gourmet, 20th Anniversary Edition. Conde' Nast Books, Random House, New York.

The New Mayo Clinic Cookbook, Eating Well for Better Health. Oxmoor House, Birmingham, AL.

Turner, Elizabeth (Editor in Chief). Vegetarian Times. El Segundo, CA.

Weil, Andrew MD, Daley, Rosie. The Healthy Kitchen, Recipes for a Better Body, Life, and Spirit. Alfred A. Knopf, New York, NY.

Whitney, Ellie, Rolfes, Sharon Rady. Understanding Nutrition. Thomson & Wadsworth. United States

APPENDIX

LivingAfterWLS Empowerment Philosophy

By Kaye Bailey

LivingAfterWLS believes that success with weight loss surgery (gastric bypass, lap band and other procedures), and in life, can be found when we focus on inner strength rather than inner weakness. As recovering morbidly obese people we have often been made to feel weak for our illness. We are not weak. We have inner resources that make us beautiful unique beings with intelligence, talent and love to share with the world. The LivingAfterWLS philosophy empowers individuals to recognize and harness their own inner strengths.

The first step to personal empowerment is personal responsibility. LivingAfterWLS holds individuals accountable for making their weight loss surgery successful. When individuals take responsibility, they feel liberated and motivated to invest personal equity in their success.

Personal empowerment is not borne of the statement "I am empowered." It is a state of mind cultivated with education, thought and validation. The LivingAfterWLS support group program and online resources are actively engaged in the pursuit of personal empowerment for all neighbors. The following core values support this philosophy:

Socialization & Culture
Social Equality
Education & Understanding
Health & Wellness
Information & Communication
Opportunity & Sustainability
LivingAfterWLS is built on the strength of relationships
　　　　LivingAfterWLS is flexible, adaptable, intelligent and creative

Overview of Metabolic & Bariatric Surgery

by American Society for Metabolic and Bariatric Surgery (2008)

I provide this report, without editing or interpretation, for your reference.

Overview: Treatment for morbid obesity and obesity-related diseases and condition; limits amount of food stomach can hold, and/or limits number of calories absorbed, by surgically reducing the stomach's capacity to a few ounces.

Candidates have a body mass index (BMI) of 40 or more, or a BMI of 35 or more with an obesity-related disease, such as Type 2 diabetes, heart disease or sleep apnea

About 220,000 people with morbid obesity in the U.S. had bariatric surgery in 2008

About 15 million people in the U.S. have morbid obesity; 1% of the clinically eligible population is being treated for morbid obesity through bariatric surgery

Bariatric surgery costs an average of $17,000 - $26,000; insurance coverage varies by provider

Impact on Obesity-Related Diseases: Can improve or resolve more than 30 obesity-related conditions, including Type 2 diabetes, heart disease, sleep apnea, hypertension and high cholesterol

- Gastric bypass resolves Type 2 diabetes in nearly 87% of patients
- Band surgery resolves Type 2 diabetes in 73% of patients
- Cuts risk of developing coronary heart disease in half
- Resolves obstructive sleep apnea in more than 85% of patients
- Bariatric Surgery: Risks vs. Benefits:
- In 2007, Federal government (Agency for Healthcare Research and Quality) and clinical studies report significant improvements in safety
- Risk of death from bariatric surgery is about 0.1%
- Bariatric surgery increases lifespan, as compared to those who do not have surgery
- Patients may improve life expectancy by 89%
- Patients may reduce their risk of premature death by 30 to 40%
- Dramatic reduction in risk of death from obesity-related diseases, as compared to those who do not have surgery
- Risk of death from diabetes down 92%, from cancer down 60% and from coronary artery disease down 56%

Long-Term Effectiveness of Bariatric Surgery:

Typically, patients have maximum weight loss within 1-2 years after surgery and maintain a substantial weight loss, with improvements in obesity-related conditions, for years afterwards

Patients may lose 30 to 50% of their excess weight 6 months after surgery and 77% of their excess weight as early as 12 months after surgery

Long-term studies show up to 10-14 years after surgery, morbidly obese patients who had surgery maintained a much greater weight loss and more favorable levels of diabetes, cholesterol and hypertension, as compared to those who did not have surgery

Adolescents and Bariatric Surgery: As obesity rates rise in the U.S., increasing number of adolescents (12-17 years old) are having bariatric surgery; an estimated 349 in 2004

Research shows that bariatric surgery may be an effective treatment for Type 2 diabetes, high blood pressure and high cholesterol in extremely obese adolescents

In November 2019 The American Academy of Pediatrics declared support of weight loss surgery in the treatment of childhood obesity under certain criteria. Their statement:

"Severe obesity among youth is an "epidemic within an epidemic" and portends a shortened life expectancy for today's children compared with those of their parents' generation. Severe obesity has outpaced less severe forms of childhood obesity in prevalence, and it disproportionately affects adolescents. Emerging evidence has linked severe obesity to the development and progression of multiple comorbid states, including increased cardiometabolic risk resulting in end-organ damage in adulthood. Lifestyle modification treatment has achieved moderate short-term success among young children and those with less severe forms of obesity, but no studies to date demonstrate significant and durable weight loss among youth with severe obesity. Metabolic and bariatric surgery has emerged as an important treatment for adults with severe obesity and, more recently, has been shown to be a safe and effective strategy for groups of youth with severe obesity."

Armstrong SC, Bolling CF, Michalsky MP, et al. AAP SECTION ON OBESITY, SECTION ON SURGERY. Pediatric Metabolic and Bariatric Surgery: Evidence, Barriers, and Best Practices. Pediatrics. 2019;144(6):e20193223

Most Common Types of Bariatric Surgery:

Gastric Bypass:

Stomach reduced from size of football to size of golf ball

Smaller stomach is attached to middle of small intestine, bypassing the section of the small intestine (duodenum) that absorbs the most calories

Patients eat less because stomach is smaller and absorb fewer calories because food does not travel through duodenum

Laparoscopic Adjustable Gastric Banding (LAGB)

Silicone band filled with saline is wrapped around upper part of stomach to create small pouch and cause restriction

Patients eat less because they feel full quickly

Size of restriction can be adjusted after surgery by adding or removing saline from band

Bilio-Pancreatic Diversion with Duodenal Switch

Similar to gastric bypass, but surgeon creates sleeve-shaped stomach

Smaller stomach is attached to final section of small intestine, bypassing the duodenum

Patients eat less because the stomach is smaller and absorb fewer calories because food does not travel through the duodenum

Newer Procedures & Surgical Devices:

Vertical Sleeve Gastrectomy

Stomach restricted by stapling and dividing it vertically, removing more than 85%

Procedure generates weight loss by restricting the amount of food that can be eaten

Currently indicated as an alternative to gastric banding

Natural Orifice Translumenal Endoscopic Surgery (NOTES)

Emerging minimally invasive procedure still in clinical trials

Surgery performed through natural orifice such as mouth or vagina, eliminating need for external incisions

Patients may experience a quicker, less painful recovery

Source: American Society for Metabolic and Bariatric Surgery. Contact: Keith Taylor (212) 527-7537. http://www.asmbs.org

Weight Loss Medications for Patients: A Review

Bariatric Times: April 1, 2018

Obesity is among the most common causes of morbidity in the United States. Few patients and providers are aware of effective treatment options for obesity besides bariatric surgery and lifestyle interventions. This review will focus on the use of medications for weight loss in patients with obesity. It will address the indications, options, costs, benefits, and effectiveness of United States Food and Drug Administration (FDA)-approved weight loss medications currently on the market.

Obesity is one of the most common causes of disability today. In the United States alone, nearly two-thirds of Americans have overweight or obesity. *Obesity is also* reaching epidemic proportions worldwide as well. Weight loss can help patients with obesity avoid suffering from such medical conditions as heart disease, diabetes, and cancer. It is critical that effective treatment options exist to help patients tackle this problem.

Obesity, however, is difficult to treat and often requires multiple therapeutic modalities. The first measures usually involve intensive lifestyle interventions, including strict diet, exercise, and cognitive changes to promote healthy eating and increased activity. Later measures can include a combination of lifestyle intervention and bariatric surgery, which is highly effective for both weight loss and control of associated comorbidities. Few other options exist for patients seeking a bridge between behavioral changes and invasive surgery. Chief among them are pharmacotherapies. Currently, there are six United States Food and Drug Administration (FDA)-approved medications for weight loss. These medicines are primarily intended either as adjuncts to diet or exercise.

Weight loss medicines have a notably checkered past. In the 1930s, dinitrophenol (DNP) gained considerable popularity for its weight-reducing effects. It works by interfering with the process that creates adenosine triphosphate (ATP). Specifically, DNP uncouples oxidative phosphorylation by increasing the basal leakage of protons across the mitochondrial membrane. This weakens the proton gradient that is necessary to fuel ATP production. The potential energy from the proton gradient is instead lost as heat. Consequently, more calories must be consumed per unit of energy produced. The medicine's weight-loss effect thus came coupled with the side effect of hyperthermia. Many patients presented with hyperthermia, cataracts, tachycardia, diaphoresis, tachypnea, and eventual cardiac arrest. By 1938, the FDA recommended against human usage of DNP.

Multiple weight loss compounds have since been studied, some of which have undergone clinical trials and been approved by the FDA for the treatment of obesity. Before prescribing any of these medications to your patients, it is important to consider the risks versus benefits of each in order to determine the safest and most effective medicine for each patient. This review addresses this critical concern in the management of the bariatric patient.

Indications: Pharmacologic therapy is indicated for any patient diagnosed with obesity (body mass index [BMI] ≥30). Some patients who are moderately overweight (BMI ≥27) but do not have obesity can use certain weight-loss drugs if they have at least one co-existing condition associated with obesity. These conditions include diabetes, hypertension, hyperlipidemia, and sleep apnea.

If the appropriate criteria are met, patients with obesity should be started on these medications when they fail to reach adequate weight loss through lifestyle intervention alone. Importantly, lifestyle intervention must continue even while patients use prescription weight loss drugs. These medicines achieve best results when used as adjuncts to a weight-loss program that is already incorporating increased exercise, behavioral therapy, and calorie-restricting diets. These medications should be discontinued if less than five percent of weight is lost in a 12-week trial.

Phentermine. First introduced in 1959, phentermine is the most commonly prescribed weight loss medication.4 It works to reduce appetite through its sympathomimetic properties. This suppression of appetite helps decrease food consumption and weight gain. A clinical trial in 2013 demonstrated that phentermine monotherapy led to at least five percent weight loss in 43 percent of patients on a low dose formulation and 46 percent on a higher dose formulation. The side effects of the drug are like those of other stimulants and include dizziness, anxiety, insomnia, tachycardia, hypertension, diarrhea, or constipation. Notably, phentermine had been historically used in tandem with an anti-obesity medication called fenfluramine that was withdrawn from the market for increasing risk of cardiac valvulopathy in patients. Most of this risk was attributed to the fenfluramine component of the drug combination, leaving phentermine available on the market. Phentermine is approved by the FDA in a lower-dose, 8mg formulation called Lomaira. It is implied that this formulation leads to similar outcomes with reduced side effects based on historical trials, which is why the FDA approved this medicine. Lomaira itself, however, has not been specifically tested in clinical trials, making these claims debatable. Phentermine is one of the more affordable weight-loss medications on the market, with an average retail price of $34.78 for 30 tablets (cost per dose: $1.16). With coupon, this medicine is available for $10.26.

Orlistat (Alli). Orlistat (marketed as Alli or Xenical) is a lipase inhibitor approved by the FDA first in 1999 as a prescription drug for obesity management and again in 2007 as an over-the-counter medication for weight loss. Orlistat achieves its effect by interrupting the absorption of fat in the gastrointestinal system. A double-blind, randomized, controlled trial in 1999 demonstrated that a third of patients who received the drug lost greater than five percent of their body weight and saw a significant drop in their serum lipid levels. The interference of fat absorption led to some predictable side effects, including fatty stools, flatulence, oily spotting, and fat-soluble vitamin deficiencies, among others.15 Orlistat is the most affordable weight-loss drug with an average retail price of $39.94 for 60 pills (cost per dose: $0.67).

Lorcaserin (Belviq). Approved in June 2012, lorcaserin (trade name Belviq) works by centrally suppressing appetite. Specifically, lorcaserin selectively activates the 5-HT2C receptors in the pro-opiomelanocortin neurons of the hypothalamus to promote satiety. In a 2010 trial, nearly 50 percent of lorcaserin-treated patients lost five percent or more of their body weight compared to only 20 percent of placebo-treated patients. Adverse effects of the drug were minimal, with most patients citing headache, dizziness, and nausea as their primary complaints. Few patients experienced the adverse cardiovascular events that less selective drugs of the serotonin class like fenfluramine caused. Belviq has an average retail price of $322.27 for 60 tablets (cost per dose: $5.37). Patients can use a free coupon to receive 13 percent off the medication, bringing the price down to $279.39.

Phentermine/topiramate (Qsymia). In July of 2012, phentermine was approved for weight loss yet again. This time, it achieved an improved therapeutic effect in combination with topiramate, an antiepileptic drug known to induce anorexia. While the exact mechanism of action is not clearly understood, the drug combination led to a significantly higher proportion of patients achieving greater than five percent weight loss compared to placebo (67% vs 17%, respectively). Drug-treated patients also saw significant reductions in hypertension and hyperlipidemia. Major adverse effects included insomnia, dry mouth, and constipation. Just as phentermine can be independently taken for weight loss, so too can topiramate. Topiramate alone can achieve the appetite suppression that Qsymia produces. This strategy should be employed when patients cannot use phentermine due to side effects or contraindications. Importantly, though, the efficacy of this drug combination reported above is specific to the Qsymia combined formulation. The effect is not as significant when phentermine and topiramate are separately prescribed but simultaneously taken. The average retail price of Qsymia is $235.94 (cost per dose: $7.86), although discounts bring the price down to $193.25. Some patients may be prescribed the components of the combination individually for a cheaper overall price, despite decreased weight-loss effectiveness.

Naltrexone/buproprion (Contrave). The naltrexone/buproprion combination drug was approved in September 2014 under the trade name Contrave. It achieved its therapeutic effect by targeting the same pro-opiomelanocortin neurons that lorcaserin acted on. Uniquely, though, the naltrexone component of Contrave antagonized opioid receptors to augment buproprion's activation of those neurons. The effect led to significantly reduced food craving and appetite suppression in patients. Approximately 56 percent of patients treated with Contrave lost greater than five percent of their weight compared to only 18 percent on placebo. The most common side effect patients reported was nausea, with minimal other adverse effects. The average retail price is $310.30 for 120 tablets (cost per dose: $2.59), but free rebates can bring the price down to $234.69.22

Liraglutide (Saxenda). Liraglutide, a GLP-1 agonist originally approved for Type 2 diabetes management, is an injectable therapy that both promotes satiety and affects glucose homeostasis. Liraglutide is produced by Novo Nordisk (Bagsværd, Denmark) in two formulations: Victoza and Saxenda. Victoza is used for glucose homeostasis in diabetes management. Saxenda is specifically indicated for weight loss. Saxenda's 3.0mg dose versus Victoza's maximum 1.8mg dose make Saxenda more effective at promoting weight loss. In 2014, the results of a double-blind, placebo-controlled trial demonstrated that 76 percent of patients on Saxenda lost greater than five percent of their weight compared to only 30 percent on placebo. Moreover, Saxenda reduced both hypertension and hyperglycemia in treated patients. Nausea and vomiting were the most common adverse effects, with the therapy being otherwise well tolerated. Saxenda for weight loss is by far the most expensive prescription weight loss medication on the market. Its average retail price is $1,405.38 for 30 injections (cost per dose: $46.85), but coupons can bring the cost down to $1,233.57 and additional rebates are also available.

Risks: In addition to the side effects of prescription weight loss drugs mentioned above, ranging from nausea to stimulant-like effects of phentermine to even the fatty stools and vitamin deficiencies caused by orlistat, there are other considerable risks of these medicines that should be kept in mind. Accordingly, patients with particular conditions that could be worsened by these side effects are contraindicated from taking those medications. Patients with cardiovascular disease, hyperthyroidism, history of drug abuse, or who are currently on monoamine oxidase inhibitors (MAOIs) or tricyclic antidepressants are recommended against using phentermine, phentermine/topiramate, or naltrexone/bupropion. Those with cholestasis or malabsorption problems should not use orlistat. Pregnant patients should avoid using all weight-loss drugs. Liraglutide is contraindicated in individuals with a family or personal history of thyroid malignancy or multiple endocrine neoplasia Type 2 (MEN2) because of its association with medullary thyroid cancer. Most of the medicines with the worst reported adverse effects have been withdrawn from the market, including sibutramine for increasing risk of cardiovascular disease, rimonabant for increasing risk of depression, and fenfluramine for increasing risk of cardiac valvulopathies and primary pulmonary hypertension.

Conclusion: Weight-loss therapeutics are important tools in obesity management. They offer auxiliary support for patients struggling to achieve their weight loss goals through diet, exercise, and behavior changes alone. Most of them help patients lose 3 to 7 percent of their excess body weight in the long term. Importantly, though, these medications are only successful when coupled with intensive lifestyle intervention. Additionally, their risks are not insignificant. Patients with certain comorbidities must be careful to avoid anti-obesity medicines that will have adverse effects on them. Given the history of hazardous drugs for weight loss, physicians are likely to be more reluctant prescribing these therapies for their patients. And although most of these medicines are reasonably priced, the more recently approved ones are less affordable. While rebates and discounts can make these drugs more affordable, patients without adequate insurance coverage might struggle to purchase them for an extended period of time.

Of the options for weight loss available to patients with obesity, lifestyle interventions remain the most safe and accessible and bariatric surgery remains the most efficacious. The reviewed medicines, while helpful as adjuncts, are not effective enough to be considered first-line. These drugs are, however, helpful for patients who do not meet the more stringent BMI criteria of 40 or 35 with comorbidities for bariatric surgery. They can also be considered for patients who need assistance with maintaining weight loss after receiving bariatric surgery, although no specific trials have been conducted to measure the efficacy of such a regimen.

With the varied risks and benefits of each of the six FDA-approved prescription and over-the-counter weight-loss medicines available today, it is important for providers to individually tailor medication regimens to their patients' unique needs. Patients with obesity remain in need of novel weight-loss therapeutics that are more effective and maintain low risk profiles.

Several new drugs not yet approved by the FDA for weight loss are being used effectively off label, including semaglutide (Ozempic). Soon, these medicines might become officially indicated for anti-obesity therapy by the FDA. As we continue to gain insights into pathophysiology of obesity, perhaps we will encounter new therapeutic targets for which drugs can be made. These efforts are essential for offering hope to patients around the world looking for assistance with managing obesity.

For article references see: Bariatric Times. 2018;15(4):8–10
http://bariatrictimes.com/weight-loss-medications-review/

Basics for Handling Food Safely

Provided by United States Department of Agriculture
Food Safety & Inspection Service
http://www.usda.gov/wps/portal/usdahome

Safe steps in food handling, cooking, and storage are essential to prevent food borne illness. You can't see, smell, or taste harmful bacteria that may cause illness

Cleanliness — Wash hands and surfaces often.

Separate — Do not cross-contaminate.

Cook — Cook to proper temperatures.

Chill — Refrigerate promptly.

Shopping:

Purchase refrigerated or frozen items after selecting your non-perishables.

Never choose meat or poultry in packaging that is torn or leaking.

Do not buy food past "Sell-By," "Use-By," or other expiration dates.

Storage

Always refrigerate perishable food within 2 hours (1 hour when the temperature is above 90 °F).

Check the temperature of your refrigerator and freezer with an appliance thermometer. The refrigerator should be at 40 °F or below and the freezer at 0 °F or below.

Cook or freeze fresh poultry, fish, ground meats, and variety meats within 2 days; other beef, veal, lamb, or pork, within 3 to 5 days.

Perishable food such as meat and poultry should be wrapped securely to maintain quality and to prevent meat juices from getting onto other food.

To maintain quality when freezing meat and poultry in its original package, wrap the package again with foil or plastic wrap that is recommended for the freezer.

In general, high-acid canned food such as tomatoes, grapefruit, and pineapple can be stored on the shelf for 12 to 18 months. Low-acid canned food such as meat, poultry, fish, and most vegetables will keep 2 to 5 years — if the can remains in good condition and has been stored in a cool, clean, and dry place. Discard cans that are dented, leaking, bulging, or rusted.

Preparation

Always wash hands with warm water and soap for 20 seconds before and after handling food.

Don't cross-contaminate. Keep raw meat, poultry, fish, and their juices away from other food. After cutting raw meats, wash cutting board, utensils, and countertops with hot, soapy water.

Cutting boards, utensils, and countertops can be sanitized by using a solution of 1 tablespoon of unscented, liquid chlorine bleach in 1 gallon of water.

Marinate meat and poultry in a covered dish in the refrigerator.

Thawing

Refrigerator: The refrigerator allows slow, safe thawing. Make sure thawing meat and poultry juices do not drip onto other food.

Cold Water: For faster thawing, place food in a leak-proof plastic bag. Submerge in cold tap water. Change the water every 30 minutes. Cook immediately after thawing.

Microwave: Cook meat and poultry immediately after microwave thawing.

Cooking

Beef, veal, and lamb steaks, roasts, and chops may be cooked to 145°F.

All uncured cuts of pork, 145°F. Cured pork should be cooked following label instructions.

Ground beef, veal and lamb to 160°F.

All poultry should reach a safe minimum internal temperature of 165°F.

Serving

Hot food should be held at 140°F or warmer.

Cold food should be held at 40°F or colder.

When serving food at a buffet, keep food hot with chafing dishes, slow cookers, and warming trays. Keep food cold by nesting dishes in bowls of ice or use small serving trays and replace them often.

Perishable food should not be left out more than 2 hours at room temperature (1 hour when the temperature is above 90 °F).

Leftovers

Discard any food left out at room temperature for more than 2 hours (1 hour if the temperature was above 90 °F).

Place food into shallow containers and immediately put in the refrigerator or freezer for rapid cooling.

Use cooked leftovers within 4 days.

About Kaye Bailey

Kaye Bailey developed the 5 Day Pouch Test in 2007 and is the owner of LivingAfterWLS and the 5 Day Pouch Test websites. Ms. Bailey, a professional research journalist, and a bariatric RNY (gastric bypass) patient since 1999, brings professional research methodology and personal experience to her publications focused on long-lasting successful weight management after surgery.

Concerned about weight regain her bariatric surgeon advised her to "get back to basics". With that vague advice Ms. Bailey says, "I read thousands of pages and conducted interviews with medical professionals including surgeons, nutritionists, and mental health providers. I collected data from WLS post-ops who honestly and generously shared their experience. My research background gave me the methodology to collect a vast amount of data. As a patient I found answers to the questions and concerns I have in common with most patients after WLS." From that the 5DPT and related works evolved.

Kaye Bailey is the author of countless articles syndicated in several languages, and books available in print and electronic format including:

The 5 Day Pouch Test Owner's Manual; Day 6: Beyond the 5 Day Pouch Test; Cooking with Kaye Methods to Meals: Protein First Recipes You Will Love; 5 Day Pouch Test Express Study Guide; 5 Day Pouch Test Complete Recipe Collection; Protein First: Understanding and Living the First Rule of WLS.

She serves as Executive Editor of the LivingAfterWLS Personal Solutions journals and planners available at Amazon and the LAWLS Bookstore. The Personal Solutions planners and journals are success promoting tools for people that believe healthy living should be a simple and painless way of life.

INDEX

RECIPE INDEX

A LIVINGAFTERWLS PUBLICATION
by Kaye Bailey
Proudly serving the healthy weight management and
weight loss surgery community since 2005.

ISBN-13: 978- 1710315042

Made in the USA
Monee, IL
27 April 2021